Airway
Management

in the Critically Ill

DATE DUE

MAY - 5 2005		JUL 2 2 2005	
APR 0 5 2017			

Airway Management

in the Critically Ill

Rade B. Vukmir, MD

The Parthenon Publishing Group

International Publishers in Medicine, Science & Technology

NEW YORK   LONDON

Library of Congress Cataloging-in-Publication Data

Airway management in the critically ill / R. Vukmir
   p.; cm.
  Includes bibliographic references and index.
  ISBN 1-84214-046-9 (alk. paper)
   1. Respiratory intensive care. 2. Airway (Medicine)
    3. Trachea–Intubation. I. Vukmir, Rade B.
  [DNLM: 1. Intubation, Intratracheal. 2. Critical
   Care. WO 280 A2978 2001]
RC735.R48 A475 2001
616.2'00428-dc21
                            00-054851

British Library Cataloguing-in-Publication Data

Airway management in the critically ill
  1. Trachea – Intubation 2. Critical care medicine
  I. Vukmir, R.B.
  617.9'6

  ISBN 1-84214-046-9

Published in the USA by
The Parthenon Publishing Group Inc.
One Blue Hill Plaza
PO Box 1564, Pearl River
New York 10965, USA

Published in the UK and Europe by
The Parthenon Publishing Group Limited
Casterton Hall, Carnforth
Lancs. LA6 2LA, UK

Copyright ©2001 The Parthenon Publishing Group

Typeset by Speedlith Photo Litho Limited, Manchester, UK
Printed and bound by Bookcraft (Bath) Ltd.,
Midsomer Norton, UK

Contents

Preface

Laryngoscopy and intubation have been described by Flagg as 'the pivot upon which turns the movement to prevent asphyxial death'. There is perhaps no area in medicine more crucial in the need to arrive at the proper endpoint than adequate airway management and control in the critically ill patient.

Perhaps more important than the process of intubation itself is the decision making that is employed to arrive at the proper strategy for airway management. This endpoint would be achieved by helping either to define that only the appropriate patient should undergo endotracheal intubation or, perhaps more importantly, to define those who should not. We are often left with the irony that the patients most in need of emergency airway control are least able to tolerate the hemodynamic and cardiopulmonary consequences of difficult or unsuccessful airway control attempts.

A patient with adequate cardiopulmonary reserve in a controlled operating room setting with adequate ventilation, preoxygenation and no anatomic barriers to intubation may often be successfully intubated after multiple attempts without sequelae. However, the critically ill patient with poor cardiopulmonary reserve accompanied by anatomic and physiological variables making intubation difficult will require a different approach and interventional strategy to prevent further physiological compromise.

Therefore, the objective of this work is to provide a structured framework to assess properly the needs of the critically ill patient in regard to emergency airway management. This can be achieved by stressing proper assessment of the routine and difficult airway, providing a successful strategy for pharmacological intervention, using alternative techniques such as adjunct and surgical airway

maneuvers and, last, evaluating long-term risks and complications of the procedure.

This book is intended to assist both the new and experienced practitioner to facilitate successful airway management in the critically ill patient. The routine intubation procedure is described for the novice and includes conventional oral and nasotracheal intubation. Pharmacological intervention to facilitate intubation is described for the intermediate practitioner. The difficult airway, surgical airway and long-term complication sections of this text are referred to the advanced practitioner. Likewise, a broad range of medical and surgical professionals that deal with airway management may benefit from reading this book. Hopefully, a balanced approach is delivered, stressing both the medical and surgical aspects of airway management relevant to anesthesia, critical care and emergency medicine, as well as medical and surgical critical care practitioners.

The first chapter provides a summary of endotracheal intubation, reviewing both the procedure and the pharmacology used in the procedure. The second chapter evaluates the management of difficult endotracheal intubation, providing predictive tools, assessment techniques and algorithms for care. The third chapter discusses the confirmation of endotracheal tube placement, which is a crucial part of the procedure. Chapter four discusses laryngotracheal injury associated with acute and prolonged intubation. The final chapter considers the surgical airway, involving cricothyroidotomy, percutaneous translaryngeal ventilation and tracheostomy, stressing approaches, complications and outcome.

Ideally after review, the practitioner will be able to use the information contained within these pages to generate his/her own intervention modes directed towards proper airway control to facilitate care in those patients who have significant cardiopulmonary compromise. Developing a standard approach to most airway emergencies will allow reliable, repetitive intervention in an emergency situation. However, the expert practitioner may need to make individual modifications according to the patient or care scenario. They may need to delineate clearly those procedures required for a routine operating suite airway control maneuver compared to a rapid sequence induction in a combative trauma patient, as well as a critically ill postoperative patient with poor cardiopulmonary reserve.

As opposed to other medical procedures and interventions, laryngoscopy is performed less often now by experienced practitioners than in the past. Chevalier Jackson described a training program for practitioners of laryngoscopy that suggested that performing approximately 100 procedures left one a beginner; after 1000 procedures you became a teacher; while 10 000 procedures defined you as a 'true expert'. In these days of multiple practitioners and subspecialists, it is often hard to achieve these lofty goals with regard to procedural experience in the direct laryngoscopy

arena. Therefore, it is even more important with less overall procedural experience that the advanced practitioner should maintain a standardized regimented approach allowing for individual modification to provide a reliable method for assessment and intervention.

My sincere appreciation goes to Christine Henderson and Melodie Braden for their tireless devotion to achieving this book's endpoint. This book is dedicated to my mother, Leni B. Vukmir, to whom I am indebted for providing the guidance and the navigation through my various educational challenges.

Rade Vukmir

Photographic credits
The author is grateful to Walter Stoy, PhD and Andrew Herlich, MD for the use of their photographic material.

Disclaimer
The recommendations in this book are meant as guidelines only and should not replace conventional care standards. In addition, drug doses should be verified for accuracy prior to administration.

Endotracheal intubation: review of procedure and pharmacology

1

INTRODUCTION

The modern clinical use of the endotracheal tube is attributed to MacEwen, who designed the device in 1880[1]. Kirstein further developed the procedure of endotracheal intubation using a direct-vision laryngoscope in 1895[2]. Common use of this technique for a variety of clinical settings was described in Jackson's 1913 work[3]. Guedel and Waters went on to develop an intratracheal catheter with an inflatable cuff to secure the airway[4].

The indications for endotracheal intubation are diverse and can be considered absolute or relative; they are modified by emergency, urgent or routine criteria based on disease severity (Table 1). Contraindications to intubation are perhaps more specific to the route – oral or nasal – than to the requirement for the procedure itself.

ANESTHESIA

The ease and success of intubation can be facilitated by the proper use of pharmacological adjunct agents. Flagg delineated the classic anesthesia sequence into: the induction period marked by excitement, rigidity and relaxation; the maintenance period; followed by the recovery phase, noting return of reflexes and level of consciousness[5]. Guedel suggested four stages of the classic ether anesthesic process: amnesia from the onset of induction to loss of consciousness with preserved pain sensation; delirium featuring uninhibited excitation, allowing an adverse response to noxious stimuli; surgical anesthesia with absence of a deleterious response to noxious stimuli; and overdosage indicated by hypotension or unreactive pupils[6].

These models illustrate the complexity of the entire anesthesia process, of which endotracheal intubation is but a small proportion. However, the significance is that attempts at intubation in a hurried unprepared fashion can be fraught with hazard. Therefore, intubation attempts without adequate premedication may result in paradoxical excitation and adverse physiological effects early in the induction phase.

These adverse effects may be avoided by a proper combination of anesthetic agents to maximize the therapeutic effect and maintain the toxic drug effect. This concept of 'balanced anesthesia' was originally described by Lundy

Table 1 Clinical use of endotracheal intubation

Indications
  anatomic difficulty
  coagulopathy (nasal)
  facial fracture (nasal)

Contraindications
Emergency
  airway obstruction
  respiratory distress
  oxygenation failure (hypoxia)
  ventilation failure (hypercarbia)
  facial trauma
  penetrating neck trauma

Urgent
  diagnostic procedures
  respiratory mechanics
  secretion clearance
  hemorrhage
  mental status alteration
  pulmonary contusion
  flail chest
  cardiac instability

Routine
  surgical intervention

in 1926[7]. The balanced anesthesia approach uses appropriate sedative agents such as benzodiazepines, analgesic agents, specifically narcotics, or hypnotic agents such as barbiturates usually combined with skeletal muscle relaxants for induction, along with inhalational agents for maintenance of anesthesia (Figure 1).

PHYSIOLOGY

Adverse physiological effects during intubation include cardiopulmonary and neurological responses to laryngeal manipulation after laryngoscopy, followed by an additional component due to passage of the endotracheal tube (ETT) itself. Most pharmacological interventions attempting to blunt the response to endotracheal intubation are directed at the cardiopulmonary system and the hemodynamic response.

Evaluation of intubation in elective surgical patients by Knight and colleagues demonstrated an increase of mean arterial pressure from baseline to 15–39% and heart rate from 12–21 beats/min, while the incidence of premature ventricular contractions was equivalent[8] (Figure 2). The adverse hemodynamic response was greater with the duration of intubation attempts from 14 to 23 s based on operator experience, as well as intubation technique[8].

The peak time to the cardiovascular response to laryngoscopy and intubation was between 26 and 31 s, with a propofol (2.5 mg/kg) induction sequence; and between 20 and 32 s with a thiopental (4.5 mg/kg) induction sequence noted in the evaluation of 30 patients by Hickey and co-workers[9]. The blood pressure response was bimodal with initial hypertension, followed by hypotension 1 min post-induction with a 2.6 (0–5.9)-kPa decrease in systolic blood pressure for propofol and 2.3 (0.4–3.8)-kPa decrease for thiopental[9]. They concluded that non-invasive hemodynamic monitoring may fail to appreciate this hypertension response.

Similar findings were reported in the cardiac population in the group of Bruder and associates of American Society of Anesthesiologists (ASA) I patients with a systemic hypertensive response to intubation,

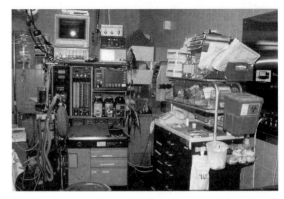

Figure 1 Anesthesia work area

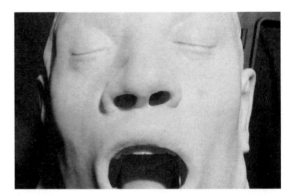

Figure 2 Laryngeal stimulus for blade insertion

with a 40–50% increase in mean arterial pressure and tachycardia with a 20% increase in heart rate beginning 1 min post-intubation for a 10-min period[10]. This population with cardiac anesthesia demonstrated myocardial ischemia secondary to sympathetic stress in 50% of the cases undergoing an induction sequence and intubation[10]. This adverse cardiac response may be monitored as an increase in rate × pressure product (RPP) equivalent to the heart rate × systolic blood pressure and is usually ≤ 125 units. Pathak and co-workers demonstrated an increase in RPP with a placebo or lidocaine (2 mg/kg, intravenously) induction sequence administered along with thiopental and succinylcholine, compared to a decrease in RPP associated with an alfentanil (15–30 mg/kg) induction sequence[11].

The effect of intubation on cardiopulmonary function has been reported by Stoelting and Peterson in a group of 36 non-cardiac patients undergoing rapid-sequence induction with morphine sulfate, scopolamine, curare, thiamylal and succinylcholine[12]. In addition to hypertension (mean arterial pressure increased by 38 mmHg) and tachycardia (increased by 25 beats/min), the arterial oxygen pressure decreased from 356 to 296 mmHg and the arterial carbon dioxide tension increased from 38 to 44 mmHg[12].

A mechanistic description of the direct laryngoscopy and somatovisceral response has been offered by Hassan and co-workers, who quantified this force as the laryngoscopy impulse (Ns) equivalent to the average force (Newtons) multiplied by the duration (seconds) of effort $(I = N \times s)$[13]. Their analysis of 40 patients suggested that the impulse directly impacts upon the hemodynamic (systolic blood pressure or heart rate) and sympathetic (serum catecholamine) response[13]. There is a biphasic response with laryngoscopy sensed by proprioceptors supplied by the glosso-pharyngeal nerve; and an additional response with vocal cord contact supplied by the superior laryngeal nerve above and the recurrent laryngeal nerve below the vocal cords, as the trachea is cannulated.

PROCEDURE

The procedural aspects of intubation are best approached in a careful, systematic fashion (Table 2). The key to success is proper assembly

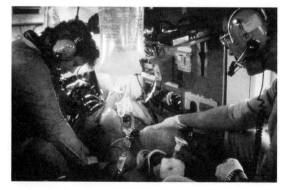

Figure 3 Emergency intubation

of equipment, clarification of indications, knowledge of pharmacology, proper procedure and a rehearsed failed intubation sequence. The route of intubation – nasal or oral – is best left to the practitioner's experience. Emergency intubation by definition involves the orotracheal route, while urgent or elective intubation can probably be achieved by nasal intubation (Table 3) (Figure 3).

The process of learning to intubate is complex, and is facilitated by planned training approaches. Stewart and co-workers examined 779 patients intubated by paramedic emergency personnel and concluded that a multimodal approach including didactic sessions, manikin training, animal models and operating room experience improved successful intubation from 77% to 94%[14]. Medical student intubation experience was examined by O'Flaherty and Adams in 30 patients; they

Table 2 Intubation procedure

(1) Equipment check-designate
(2) Preoxygenation (facemask – 15 l/min)
      Pulse oximetry
(3) Ventilation (as necessary)
      Suction, airway
      Mask ventilation
      Cricoid pressure
(4) Venous access, fluid
(5) Equipment check
      Endotracheal tube, lubricant, stylet
      Position
      Suction
(6) Indication
      Reversible causes
      Absolute–emergency–relative
(7) Route–operator expertise
(8) Intubation
      Awake – topical anesthesia
      Sedation – benzodiazepine, narcotic
      Rapid sequence – muscle relaxant
(9) Confirmation
         visualization
            end-tidal CO_2 partial pressure, chest X-ray
         auscultation, oximetry
         release cricoid pressure
(10) Failed intubation
         help, bag valve mask ventilation
            re-evaluate, second attempt
(11) Second operator
(12) Surgical airway
         percutaneous cricothyroid jet
         conventional

demonstrated a 33% likelihood of success on the first attempt, with only slightly over half (53%) correctly confirmed. The intubation success rate had improved to 93% by the third attempt, but there was little improvement in the ability to confirm the endotracheal tube position[15].

Difficult intubation training scenarios for anesthesia trainees evaluated by Goldberg and co-workers in 40 patients found no difference in patient stability or the monitoring of cardiopulmonary variables – heart rate, blood pressure and oxygen saturation – but yielded a 25% esophageal intubation rate[16]. Instruction in this airway skill requires careful didactics, structured experience and healthy respect for a potentially lethal intervention for patient care.

PHARMACOLOGY

Proper intubation technique requires appropriate knowledge and experience in the use of pharmacological agents. The array of drugs used to facilitate intubation should be combined to maximize the therapeutic effect, while minimizing the adverse response during the induction sequence (Table 4).

Conventional methods of intubation, including nasotracheal and awake intubation, are facilitated by the use of local anesthetic agents, while direct orotracheal intubation is assisted by the use of sedative and relaxant regimens (Figures 4–9).

LOCAL ANESTHETICS

The use of local anesthesia to facilitate the intubation procedure was established in the early 20th century. Koller published a treatise on the attributes of the local anesthetic technique including the use of cocaine as a topical agent[17]. Knoefel and associates described the use of vasoconstrictor agents to prevent acute intoxication from local anesthetic agents[18].

Table 3 Route of intubation

Nasal	Oral
Indications	
Operator expertise	Operator expertise
Spontaneous respiration	Absent respiration
Comfortable maintenance	Comfortable induction
Contraindications	
Coagulopathy	Anatomic difficulty
Facial fracture	
Neutropenia	
Thrombocytopenia	
Disadvantages	
Sinusitis	Dental trauma
Preparation time	Cervical spine movement

Table 4 Pharmacological agents used to facilitate intubation

	Autonomic blockade	Amnesia	Analgesia	Anxiolysis	Dissociation	Hypnosis	Sedation	Relaxation
Local anesthetics								
topical			+					
intravenous			+					
Neuroleptics		+		.	+		+	
Hypnotics		+		.		+		
Adrenergic antagonists							+	
beta	+							
alpha	+							
Anticholinergic	+							
Benzodiazepines		+						
Narcotics	+		+	+			+	
Anesthetics			+	+	+	+	+	
intravenous								
inhalational								
Neuromuscular blocking agents (NMBAs)								+

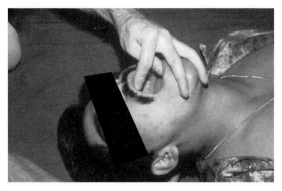

Figure 4   Scissors mouth opening procedure

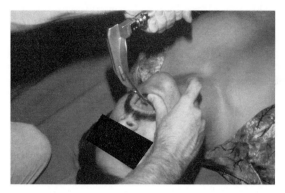

Figure 5   Careful blade insertion

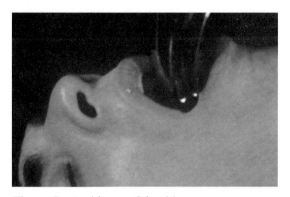

Figure 6   Avoidance of dentition

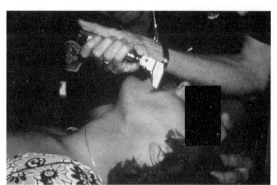

Figure 7   Lift, don't lever, avoiding the use of the teeth as a fulcrum

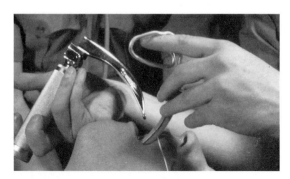

Figure 8   Careful blade removal

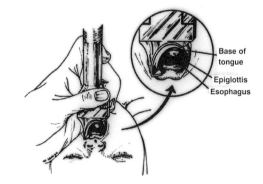

Figure 9   Oropharynx and vocal cords

The local anesthetics may be classified into two groups, based on chemical structure. The amide-based compounds include lidocaine, mepivacaine, bupivacaine, etidocaine and prilocaine, which are administered by an intravenous route and are degraded by the hepatic microsomal enzyme system. The ester-based compounds include procaine, tetracaine, cocaine and benzocaine, which may be administered by a topical route and are metabolized by the plasma cholinesterase system. The incidence of allergic reactions is much higher for the ester compared to the amide agents.

The most commonly used amide agent is lidocaine administered by the topical route in concentrations of 4% (40 mg/ml) and 10% (10 mg/ml) or the intravenous route in concentrations of 1% (10 mg/ml) and 2% (20 mg/ml). Doses of 3.5 mg/kg or a total of 300 mg are usually associated with significant toxicity, with serum levels of > 4–6.0 μg/dl, and patients are more sensitive if hepatic degradation or renal excretion is decreased during illness.

The addition of a vasoconstricting agent such as epinephrine (adrenaline) potentiates the effects of local anesthesia while minimizing toxicity. The most commonly employed mixture for topical or nerve block use is 1% lidocaine with 1 : 200 000 epinephrine, dispensed as a 30-ml vial containing 10 mg/ml of lidocaine or 300 mg, and 0.01 mg/ml (10 μg/ml) of epinephrine or 300 mg unit dose. The addition of a vasoconstrictor allows administration of a maximum dose of 7 mg/kg or a total of 500 mg of lidocaine with epinephrine. This local anesthetic–vasoconstrictor combination is seldom used in the intubation setting, owing to concerns of systemic absorption from vascular beds.

The use of topical cocaine mixtures – 4% (40 mg/ml) or 10% (100 mg/ml) – is the standard for topical vasoconstriction and anesthesia for nasal intubation. However, this compound is not commonly employed, owing to difficulty with availability and a narrow therapeutic range, with toxicity occurring when as little as 20 mg has been administered, and over 1 g is a lethal dose.

Nasal intubation was first described by Magill in 1928, using a blind technique with carbon dioxide as a respiratory stimulant to facilitate ETT passage[19]. The proper procedure requires adequate preparation including topical vasoconstriction using phenylephrine 0.5% or oxymetazoline 0.05% followed by lidocaine 2% viscous lubricant. Sometimes, significant complications are encountered including epistaxis, septum or turbinate trauma, polypectomy or retropharyngeal perforation[20] (Figures 10–14).

Hartigan and co-workers performed a clinical trial of anesthesia for blind nasotracheal intubation in 100 patients, comparing the control, lidocaine 1.5 mg/kg intravenously, phenylephrine 0.2 mg of 0.25% each nostril, and lidocaine 30 mg of 10% each nostril, after a thiopentone 4-mg/kg induction sequence. The best tolerated regimen, measured as blunting of the mean arterial pressure rise, was topical lidocaine, followed by moderate elevation with topical phenylephrine or the control, with a sustained hypertensive response noted with intravenous lidocaine[21].

Clinical evaluation suggested a 65% success rate for nasal intubation in a trial by Dronen and colleagues of 52 overdose patients, comparing succinylcholine-assisted oral intubation requiring increased procedural time (4.6–1.0 min), number of attempts (3.7–1.3) and complication rates, with epistaxis in 69%, emesis in 17% and aspiration in 10%[22] of the nasal groups. This success rate in the emergency patient was improved to 96% in Fassolt's trial of modified nasal intubation with the administration of a muscle relaxant in a controlled operative setting[23]. Pharmacological intervention, topical vasoconstriction and local anesthesia, perhaps followed by sedation, are endorsed for the emergency or urgent case, whereas muscle relaxant-assisted procedures are not recommended for novice practitioners.

Awake intubation uses local anesthesia, allowing analgesia, while maintaining airway protective reflexes. Thomas reported a 100% success rate in a group of 25 critically ill, elderly, or anticipated difficult intubation patients[24]. Lee and co-workers described 30 high-risk adult patients who underwent successful intubation after transtracheal nerve block with no change in hemodynamics or oxygen saturation[25]. However, the difficult airway patient is often more unstable than the elective patient, manifesting hypoxemia, hypercarbia and acidosis associated with sedative administration, stressing the importance of supplemental oxygen administration and close monitoring[26].

Another airway option is the use of nasal fiberoptic-assisted intubation. Hawkyard and colleagues compared awake fiberoptic-assisted intubation with oral intubation under general anesthesia, noting a blunted hypertensive (mean arterial pressure 9–35 mmHg) and tachycardiac response (heart rate 3–24 beats/min) to intubation[27].

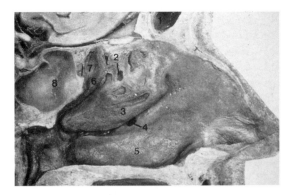

Figure 10   Cross-section of the nasopharynx

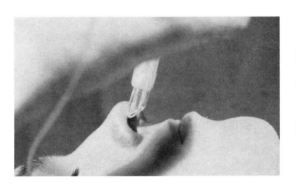

Figure 11   Lateral ETT alignment

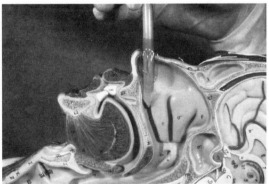

Figure 12   ETT bevel between nasal conchae

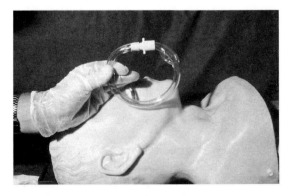

Figure 13   Increasing ETT curvature

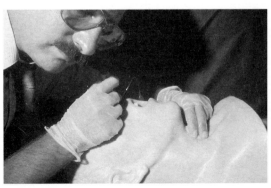

Figure 14   Auscultation for successful placement

The efficacy of various routes of local anesthetic administration – topical, aerosolized, intravenous or local injection – have been evaluated. Often a staged approach incorporating a combination of techniques is used for awake intubation. The posterior pharynx can be topically anesthetized with 10% xylocaine, which is associated with a decreased allergic or adverse reaction rate compared to benzocaine, which is associated with a particulate sensation in patients. The superior laryngeal nerve responsible for sensation above the vocal cords is approached via a transmucosal route where a pledget of 4% lidocaine is applied to the pyriform fossa by Krause's forceps[28]. Care should be used to minimize systemic absorption.

Invasive approaches include local injection of the glossopharyngeal nerve responsible for oropharyngeal sensation at the palatoglossal fold. The recurrent laryngeal nerve supplying the area below the vocal cords is approached from an external angle just inferior to the lateral thyroid cartilage. Lastly, the transtracheal area can be anesthetized by cricothyroid membrane puncture using a 25-gauge needle and 2–4 ml of 2% lidocaine, especially helpful for bronchoscopic approaches.

Stoelting studied 36 patients, comparing lidocaine administered by laryngotracheal anesthetic injection (2 mg/kg), the viscous (2.5 ml of 2%) or the intravenous (1.5 mg/kg) routes[29]. The incidence of an adverse hemodynamic response was greater with topical (11 of 12) compared with viscous (six of 12) or intravenous (four of 12) lidocaine, and the extent of the rise was 40, 27 and 21 mm/kg, respectively[29]. He concluded that local administration of viscous lidocaine was helpful, whereas intravenous lidocaine was associated with significant central nervous system (CNS) depression.

Derbyshire and co-workers compared typical lidocaine regimens in 30 elective gynecological patients including 4% spray (160 mg), 4% laryngotracheal anesthetic (160 mg) or normal saline control[30]. They concluded that the response to intubation including an increase in mean arterial pressure, heart rate, plasma epinephrine and norepinephrine levels began at 1 min post-intubation and had resolved by 5 min, and was not prevented by any topical regimen studied[30].

The neurosurgical population, specifically 22 brain tumor patients, was evaluated by Hamill and associates, who compared laryngotracheal anesthetic lidocaine (4 ml of 4%) and intravenous lidocaine (1.5 mg/kg)[31]. They reported that intravenous lidocaine was more effective at blunting an adverse response to intubation, measured as an increase in mean arterial pressure, heart rate and intracranial pressure[31]. However, Denlinger and co-workers found that protection was afforded to the cardiac patient receiving topical administration of 3 ml of 4% lidocaine compared to saline placebo from the hypertensive rise (13 to 39 mmHg) seen with intubation[32].

The use of intravenous lidocaine (1.5 mg/kg) was compared with control conditions during the induction sequence in 16 gynecological patients reported by Chraemmer-Jorgensen and colleagues[33]. They found no difference with lidocaine pretreatment 2 min prior to intubation with significant increases in mean arterial pressure (46%) and heart rate (57%) and a decrease in left ventricular ejection fraction (60–40%)[33].

Alternative methods of lidocaine administration include nebulization described by Abou-Madi and associates, where a 3.5–7-mg/kg dose was administered via an aerosolized route in 20 patients[34]. There was significant protection in the treatment group preventing an increase in systolic blood pressure (10% to 56%), heart rate (16% to 39%) or arrythmia incidence (0% to 40%) compared to control groups[34].

Lastly, anesthesia below the level of the vocal cords innervated by the recurrent laryngeal nerve may be achieved by cricothyroid puncture and subglottic lidocaine administration. Boster and colleagues described the use of the transtracheal anesthetic technique in seven comatose patients[35]. This technique required topical administration of a significant amount (5.67 ± 1.2 mg/kg) of lidocaine and required prolonged time to onset (5.1 ± 3.2 min) with maximal effect achieved at 18.7 ± 8.7 min[35]. This technique may be of benefit when used as adjunct therapy in awake intubation, utilizing much smaller doses (2–4 ml) of 4% lidocaine administration by cricothyroid membrane puncture with a 25-gauge needle and syringe (Figure 15).

The use of the local anesthetic technique to facilitate awake oral and nasal intubation strategies has some efficacy, although this is not conclusive, and should be considered to be based on the experience of the operator.

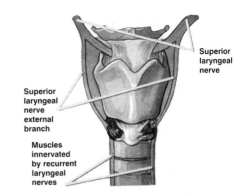

Figure 15   Superior and recurrent laryngeal nerve

Aspiration precautions

Optimal preparation for intubation includes adequate monitoring and preoxygenation. Ideally, the patient should have a cardiac monitor, pulse oximetry and capnography available. A prospective study of 191 patients monitored with continuous pulse oximetry suggested a 22% rate of desaturation (< 90%) in the monitoring group, compared to 13.5% in the unmonitored group, but the latter was associated with a more significant duration of significant desaturation (< 85%)[36].

Preoxygenation with an increased inspired oxygen concentration (FiO_2 100%) for adequate duration (4–8 min) increases the amount of oxygen bound to hemoglobin, creating a margin of safety during intubation attempts. This margin of safety is decreased in those in an emergency, chronically ill or with an inadequate duration of preoxygenation. An alternative preoxygenation technique that has been suggested is a strategy with shorter duration and maximal inhalation. Gambee and co-workers evaluated 12 patients and compared hyperventilation for 3 min and four maximal inspiration breaths. There was less desaturation in the hyperventilation group taking 7.9 vs. 5.6 min to reach 97% arterial saturation followed by 8.9 vs. 6.8 min for 90% saturation[37].

The use of cricoid pressure to prevent gastric insufflation or regurgitation during active ventilation was described in resuscitation studies of the late 1800s and more recently by Sellick in 1961[38]. This maneuver required digital posterior compression of the cricoid ring effectively closing the esophagus. The Sellick maneuver was intended to prevent aspiration of gastric contents. The additional benefit of decreasing gastric insufflation was proven by Petito and Russell in a prospective trial of mask ventilation in conjunction with cricoid pressure, revealing a significant decrease in intragastric gas measured in the treatment group[39].

The sequelae of gastric aspiration are significant, resulting in a 25% mortality reported in Mendelson's description of the classic clinical syndrome occurring in obstetric patients undergoing anesthesia in 1946[40]. The use of pharmacological intervention (non-particulate antacids acutely, and histamine-2 antagonists electively) has been shown to decrease the acid component of aspiration damage.

The non-particulate antacids available include sodium citrate with pH 4.5, administered in a 30-ml dose with onset in 10–60 min; potassium citrate with pH 5.2, administered in a 15-ml dose with onset in 10–45 min; and sodium bicarbonate with pH 7.5, administered in a 5-ml dose with onset in 10 min. Dewan and co-workers studied the use of sodium bicarbonate in cervical section patients, with a pH of 2.29 ± 1.77, who improved after administration with an unchanged gastric volume[41].

The histamine-2 antagonists are used with less emergency need for intubation. Popat and colleagues compared prophylactic histamine-2 antagonists in 90 elective gynecological patients demonstrating a gastric pH of < 2.5 in 7% of those administered nizatidine, 20% with ranitidine and 68% with placebo; the residual volume was similar in all groups[42]. Suojaranta-Ylinen and associates evaluated 114 general surgery patients comparing famotidine (40 mg), ranitidine (300 mg) and sodium citrate (30 ml), demonstrating increased pH in all cases with a decreased intragastric volume in all but the last[43]. Thus, the non-particulate antacids are equally effective, act more rapidly with the potential disadvantage of increasing gastric volume, but are better suited to emergency indications than are histamine-2 antagonists.

Premedication

The administration of medications to assist in the tolerance of painful procedures has many historical references. Wren discussed the intravenous administration of sedatives in 'An account of the rise and attempts of a way to convey liquors immediately into the mass of blood' in 1665[44].

The neuroleptic class may be used in conscious sedation protocols, which emphasize adequate physician supervision and cardiopulmonary monitoring in an attempt to avoid intubation. Droperidol is a major tranquilizer administered in a 1.25–5.0-mg intravenous dose or a 2.5–10.0-mg intramuscular dose with a 5–10-min onset of action and hepatic degradation followed by renal excretion. The effect is described as 'psychological indifference' to the environment, but it can be associated with paradoxical agitation or extrapyramidal effects of hypotension due to α-receptor antagonism. Thomas and colleagues performed a study comparing droperidol (5 mg) and haloperidol (5 mg), finding that the former agent was superior by the intramuscular route and equivalent by the intravenous route, with minimal side-effects[45].

Pharmacological agents that have a hypnotic effect, such as chloral-based compounds, were described for use in anesthesia by Oré in 1872[46].

Greenberg and co-workers described their clinical use with a dose of 50 mg/kg providing sedation, while a dose of 100 mg/kg (maximum 2000 mg) provided a hypnotic effect with a 7% rate of adverse effects, mainly gastrointestinal symptoms or oversedation[47]. Rumm and associates found chloral hydrate 86% successful in pediatric sedation, and noted failure in those who were neurologically impaired[48].

Cardiovascular sequelae

The induction sequence for intubation is often met with significant cardiovascular sequelae such as dysrhythmia or blood pressure abnormalities. Proper use must be made of anticholinergic drugs, adrenergic antagonists and other cardioprotective agents. It is essential to identify those patients at risk for cardiovascular complications during the intubation induction sequence. However, it is crucial that adequate sedation is administered prior to intubation, before considering a cardioprotective agent.

Anticholinergic agents may be utilized to prevent significant bradycardia after vagal stimulation during intubation. Commonly used agents include atropine (0.4 mg, intravenously), glycopyrrolate (0.2 mg, intravenously) or scopolamine (0.1 mg, intravenously) administered to a normal adult. Mirakhur and Dundee compared these agents and found the incidence of dysrhythmia greater for atropine and scopolamine, followed by glycopyrrolate compared to control; the incidence of hemodynamic side-effects including hypotension and bradycardia was similar[49]. Braunn and colleagues evaluated the use of anticholinergic agents in 100 ASA I/II patients targeting the oculocardiac bradycardiac reflex in ophthalmological surgery. They compared atropine (10 μg/kg) with glycopyrrolate (5 μg/kg) and found no difference when these were administered prophylactically to prevent arrhythmia or bradycardia[50]. Therefore, it would not seem prudent to administer these prophylactically to adult patients and to use them therapeutically in pediatric patients, where this side-effect is more pronounced.

Sympathetic antagonists are most commonly used to blunt the response after the catecholamine surge due to laryngoscopy in specific populations at risk, including those with significant ischemia or head injury. Esmolol is often used in the acute care setting. This cardioselective agent has poor lipid solubility and minimal intrinsic sympathetic activity, resulting in a short-acting agent with a half-life of 9 min, protective of a catecholamine-sensitized heart. The drug administration strategy is complex: a loading dose of 50 μg/kg per min is administered incrementally to a total of 500 μg/kg per min followed by a continuous infusion of 25–50 μg/kg per min[51]. However, even with a careful dosing strategy, myocardial depression and hypotension can occur.

Helfman and associates evaluated ASA grade II–IV patients who underwent induction with thiopental, succinylcholine and isoflurane along with esmolol (150 mg), lidocaine (200 mg) and fentanyl (200 μg)[51]. An average adverse hemodynamic response of a 44% increase in heart rate and a 36% decrease in systolic blood pressure with laryngoscopy was reduced with esmolol, but not with fentanyl or lidocaine. Kovac and colleagues administered a large esmolol bolus (1.5 mg/kg) prior to intubation, demonstrating a stable heart rate, but an increase in mean arterial pressure and intraocular pressure[52].

A prospective double-blind evaluation was carried out of esmolol administered as 500 μg/kg over 4 min and 300 μg/kg over 8 min compared to placebo and found a 50% decrease in heart rate, RPP, systolic arterial pressure and mean arterial pressure after intubation[53]. The combination of esmolol (1 mg/kg) and fentanyl (2 μg/kg) was more effective with the former blocking tachycardia, and the latter blunting the hypertensive response compared to either drug alone or placebo, based on the trial of 44 patients by Gaubatz and Wehner[54].

Additional cardioactive agents that may be used in the intubation sequence include α-antagonists or coronary vasodilators. Labetalol, a combined α_1, non-selective β-antagonist, was administered in a 5–10-mg dose and compared

with lidocaine (100 mg) or placebo in the controlled, randomized, blinded trial of 40 patients by Inada and associates, controlling heart rate but not hypertension after intubation[55]. Dahlgren and co-workers evaluated the effects of nitroglycerine (4 μg/kg bolus, or 1 μg/kg infusion), lidocaine and propranolol (0.01 mg/kg) given before induction of 35 patients undergoing coronary artery bypass graft (CABG)[56]. The administration of a nitroglycerine bolus and topical lidocaine was effective in minimizing the decreased ejection fraction or increased end-diastolic volume with laryngoscopy[56].

Thus, the most effective agents for blunting an adverse response are narcotic analgesics for emergency cases, and sympathetic antagonists in cardiac patients (Table 5).

Benzodiazepines

Sedation is the process of attenuation of excessive reactions to noxious stimuli[57]. Avoidance of intoxication can be achieved by using smaller amounts of neuromodulators, combined into a 'lytic cocktail', which has a destructuring effect on organized neural transmission. Benzodiazepines were first described for use as psychotherapeutic agents by Randall and colleagues in 1961[58]. Their use in anesthesia induction sequences as

Table 5 Cardioprotective agents during intubation

	Efficacy
Emergency cases	
Narcotic fentanyl	++
β-Antagonist esmolol	++
Local anesthetic lidocaine	+/–
Elective cardiac cases	
Coronary vasodilator nitroglycerine	+
Central agonist clonidine	+
Calcium antagonist nifedipine	+
α-Antagonist	–

hypnotic agents was reported by Huguenard and Deligne[59] and Douit[60] in 1965.

Diazepam was used in a 0.05–0.1-mg/kg intravenous dose with rapid onset of amnesia, often with prolonged (15 min to 3 h) duration. Although the drug was an effective sedative, adverse effects of hypotension and vascular irritation initiated a search for additional agents.

Diazepam has proven both safe and effective in this setting. Samuelson and associates evaluated 30 patients with ischemic heart disease, comparing diazepam (0.5 mg/kg) and midazolam (0.2 mg/kg)[61]. They demonstrated that diazepam decreased systolic blood pressure, while midazolam decreased systolic arterial pressure, pulmonary artery pressure, pulmonary artery occlusion pressure, stroke index (SI), and right and left ventricular stroke work index (RVSWI, LVSWI) and concluded that midazolam was associated with significant cardiovascular compromise[61].

However, Tateishi and colleagues suggested that the administration of diazepam (0.25 mg/kg) to neurosurgical patients with elevated intracranial pressure (> 15 mmHg) resulted in significant hemodynamic instability with a decrease in mean arterial pressure of 82%, and cerebral perfusion pressure of 77%[62].

Lorazepam has been administered in a 0.05-mg/kg intravenous dose with onset of action within 5–10 min with duration of 4–6 h. This benzodiazepine is highly lipophilic with complete amnesia obtained for intubation, and only occasional paradoxical CNS excitation noted[63].

Currently, the most commonly used benzodiazepine for an induction sequence is midazolam. The advantages of this agent, administered in a dose of 0.03–0.08 mg/kg, are its rapid onset of action (1–3 min) and shorter duration (1–2 h) of effect. Beneficial effects include effective amnesia, with only occasional hypotension noted.

Sievers and associates examined midazolam as a conscious sedation agent in pediatrics, noting effective amnesia in 90% but with significant hypoxemia (oxygen saturation ≤ 90%) in 13% of cases[64]. Wright and co-workers evaluated 389 patients administered midazolam at a mean dose of 3.8 mg (0.5–2.0 mg) for sedation. Complications were minimal (1.0%) with side-effects including respiratory depression (0.5%) and hypotension (0.5%), which seemed to occur more commonly (7%) with concurrent narcotic administration[65]. Bailey and colleagues retrospectively evaluated 80 cases of anesthetic death where midazolam had been administered, and found that 78% were felt to be respiratory in nature and 57% associated with narcotic use, and 77 of 80 patients suffered arrest while unattended[66].

A clinical trial of rapid sequence induction regimens comparing midazolam (0.2 mg/kg) and fentanyl (50 μg) versus thiamylal (4 mg/kg) suggested equivalent intubating conditions including time of onset for all agents[67]. In addition, there was less hemodynamic depression and a decreased anesthetic requirement.

Narcotics

Narcotic analgesics were administered by the intravenous route to induce anesthesia in early cases of operative intervention. Bartholow described the use of hypodermic medications in 1873, and Brederfeld reported the use of intravenous morphine as an anesthesia adjunct in 1916[68,69].

Fentanyl is the most widely used narcotic agent for an intubation induction sequence. Fentanyl has an equipotency of 10× the morphine dose, estimated from the actual potency of a 100× increase factored against an ultrashort half-life, resulting in a reduced equivalent effect. The induction dose is 1–5 μg/kg by the intravenous route with both onset and half-life in the range of 1–2 min. The drug's main effects include analgesia with only minimal amnesia, but slight CNS depression due to lipid solubility. The most common side-effects are respiratory depression, hypotension, bradycardia and 'chest wall rigidity' occurring infrequently, in less than 1 in 1000 cases.

The conscious sedation protocol suggests a procedural dose of 180 μg with a range of 25–1400 μg intravenously, with respiratory depression in 0.7% and hypotension in 0.4% of patients, noting synergism with midazolam, haloperidol or alcohol[70]. From and co-workers evaluated the efficacy of sufentanil (1 μg/kg load followed by 0.3 μg/kg per h) and alfentanil (75 μg/kg, 33.5 μg/kg per h) noting increased hypotension with alfentanil and respiratory depression with sufentanil[71].

Induction sequences were examined by Saltanov and colleagues in 132 patients, comparing thiopental (4–5 mg/kg), thiopental and fentanyl (1.5 μg/kg), thiopental and topical lidocaine (10%), propofol (4–5 μg/kg) and fentanyl (1.5 μg/kg), thiopental and fentanyl (3 μg/kg), and diazepam (1.5–2.0 mg) and fentanyl (3–5 μg/kg)[72]. They concluded that adequate analgesia with higher-dose fentanyl (3–5 μg/kg) was the most effective component of the induction sequence, prohibiting cardiovascular side-effects, and also stressed the monitoring of adequate intravascular volume, often requiring fluid loading.

Cardiovascular side-effects during laryngoscopy were compared between a thiopental (5 mg/kg) control group associated with a 34% increase in heart rate, 23% increase in mean arterial pressure and 147% increase in basal norepinephrine level during intubation, and groups treated with fentanyl (6 μg/kg) and with thiopental and midazolam (0.2 mg/kg); fentanyl was associated with improved efficacy of the narcotic component[73]. Chraemmer-Jorgensen and associates concluded that the combination of midazolam and fentanyl was equivalent to the barbiturate induction sequence, with the adverse cardiovascular effects minimized by the narcotic while providing equivalent intubating conditions[73].

The midazolam and fentanyl induction sequence reported by Bailey and co-workers in 12 patients also suggested that respiratory depression did not occur with the use of midazolam alone, while hypoxemia and hypercarbia occurred in 50% (six) of the fentanyl cases. The combination of midazolam and fentanyl caused apnea and hypercarbia in 50% (six) of the cases and hypoxemia in 91% (11) of patients[66].

Therefore, the combination of midazolam providing amnesia and fentanyl providing cardiovascular protection is effective, although the incidence of adverse cardiopulmonary effects is noteworthy.

Barbiturates

The induction of anesthesia by intravenous injection of sodium-iso-amyl-ethyl barbiturate was reported in 1929 by Zerfas and colleagues[74]. This report was followed in the same year by that of Lundy, describing the use of barbiturates in 1000 surgical cases, as anesthetic or hypnotic agents[75]. Later, in 1935, he reported the use of sodium pentothal as an intravenous anesthetic agent[76].

Thiopental is the prototypical barbiturate amnestic induction agent administered in an intravenous dose of 1–4 mg/kg, with onset in 30 s and 10–15-min duration of action. Adverse effects include systemic hypotension, myocardial depression, and decreased cerebral blood flow and intracranial pressure.

Giffin and co-workers compared thiopental (2.7 mg/kg) with midazolam (0.2 mg/kg) as the amnestic agent used in intubation and induction in 17 brain tumor patients[77]. They reported a rapid onset until intubating conditions (1.0 vs. 2.5 min) with thiopental, while midazolam caused tachycardia but with better regulation of cerebral perfusion pressure, but otherwise no difference between the drugs[77]. Alvarez Gomez and colleagues compared thiopental (5.0 mg/kg) with midazolam (0.3 mg/kg) in 50 patients, evaluating the effect on muscle relaxation. Both agents provided equivalent intubating conditions measured as onset of effect, maximum blockade, duration of clinical response and spontaneous recovery index[78].

Caution is certainly warranted in the critically ill, with significant hemodynamic compromise occasionally resulting in cardiac arrest. First reported in 1945 after its use in World War II casualties in the South Pacific, it was concluded that thiopental was an agent better suited for euthanasia than induction.

Methohexital is more commonly used for sedation than for induction. Zink and associates administered a dose of 1.6 mg/kg resulting in minor (-1.8 ± 2.0 mmHg systolic blood pressure) hemodynamic alterations in 17.6% of 102 patients[79].

INTRAVENOUS ANESTHETICS

The use of dissociative anesthetic agents, decreasing both the cognitive awareness and the discomfort of intubation, has been described as a part of an induction sequence or as a single agent. Ketamine is a dissociative anesthetic administered in an intravenous dose of 1–2 mg/kg or intramuscular dose of 3–5 mg/kg with rapid onset (2–3 min) and duration (5–10 min) of action. Ketamine provides somatic analgesia and blocks cerebral association pathways in the absence of hypotension commonly found with other amnestic agents. Adverse side-effects include hypertension and tachycardia, quantified as an increase in RPP, bronchorrhea due to muscarinic receptor activation, and increased cerebral blood flow, intracranial pressure and cerebral metabolic rate of oxygen consumption ($CMRO_2$).

Perhaps the optimal use of this drug is for patients in whom intravenous access cannot be obtained and an intramuscular route is used, such as trauma or pediatric patients. Ketamine may also be beneficial in the hypotensive, although it is contraindicated in trauma with concomitant head injury or in those with cardiac ischemia. The drug also finds utility as an induction agent in those with limited mental facilities unable to understand the need for intravenous access. Kruger and Benad described the additional benefit of bronchodilatation in 16 of 24 asthmatic patients when ketamine (3.5 mg/kg) was used therapeutically[80]. There may be a dual benefit of use in the intubation of those with severe asthma, where intubation alone often does not reverse the primary condition.

However, most discussion concerns adverse side-effects. White and colleagues described sensory misperception involving the inferior colliculus–acoustic relay and medical geniculate nucleus–visual relay with post-anesthesia emergence occurring in 12% of patients[81].

Cartwright and Pingel compared midazolam (0.07 mg/kg) to diazepam (0.12 mg/kg) observing emergency phenomena, and found a decrease (27% to 7%) with midazolam[82]. Recently, the effect on intracranial hemodynamics was re-examined. Pfenninger and co-workers used a porcine epidural compression model to illustrate that, with normal systemic arterial pressure, there was minimal intracranial pressure change; in the hypotensive state, the decrease in cerebral perfusion was due to the decrease in mean arterial pressure as much as to an increase in intracranial pressure[83].

Propofol has been used for induction as well as sedation. This non-opioid anesthetic agent is administered in a 1.5–2.5-mg/kg bolus dose with onset of 1–2 min and duration of 30 min. The major side-effect is hypotension, but slightly lessened compared to that of other commonly used agents.

Paulin and associates examined the use of propofol in 20 elective abdominal aortic aneurysm repair patients with coronary artery disease[84]. Adverse effects included a decrease in systolic blood pressure (17%), cardiac output (12%) and systemic vascular resistance (7%) with stable heart rate, with favorable effects noted on myocardial oxygen consumption. Coley and co-workers compared propofol (2.25 mg/kg) with thiopental (4.8 mg/kg) in 48 patients, and noted adverse hemodynamic effects in 100% of patients[85]. The hypotension was greater for propofol, dose related and proportional to ASA status.

Etomidate is associated with the most hemodynamic stability of all induction agents. This ultrashort benzylimidazole sedative–hypnotic agent is administered in a dose of 0.1–0.4 mg/kg with onset in 30–60 s and a duration of 3–5 min. Hypotension can occur in a dose-related fashion, usually in the most critically ill patients. Side-effects include nausea, myoclonus, myalgia and adrenal suppression due to decreased steroidogenesis, as well as decreased cerebral blood flow and intracranial pressure.

Early work suggested that etomidate had 25× the potency and 6× the therapeutic index of sodium thiopental[86]. The drug had a distribution time of 2.81 ± 1.64 min, elimination time of 3.88 ± 1.11 h and clearance of 954 ± 178 ml/min and was felt to have a cerebral protective effect, decreasing cerebral blood flow, intracranial pressure and $CMRO_2$[86]. Giese and co-workers compared etomidate (0.4 mg/kg) with thiopental (4 mg/kg) in 83 ASA I/II patients[87]. Both drugs were found to blunt the tachycardiac response and increase systolic blood pressure with similar rates of nausea and vomiting, while etomidate was associated with myoclonus and thiopental was associated with apnea.

Thomas and colleagues evaluated etomidate and methohexital in 45 cardiac surgery patients[88]. Etomidate was found to have no effect on blood pressure during induction, and an increase in systolic blood pressure (36%) and heart rate (41%) and a decrease in SI (21%) during intubation, but the SI (32%) returned to normal post-intubation. Methohexital produced more significant vasodilatation, myocardial depression and tachycardia.

INHALATIONAL ANESTHETICS

The use of inhalational agents antedated the intravenous route for administration of anesthesia. Early reports were by Snow in 1847 describing ether anesthesia, Worthington in 1848 describing chloroform anesthesia and Hewitt in 1887 describing the combination between ether and nitrous oxide[89–91]. Modern

anesthetic practice involved the use of cyclo-propane as the volatile anesthetic agent reported by Stiles and colleagues in 1934[92].

Inhalational agents have been used for induction for those without intravenous access, such as pediatric or emergency cases. The volatile agents are summarized in Table 6[93]. Halothane is often used in pediatrics, or in those with asthma or secondary bronchospasm. Isoflurane may be used for emergency induction in adult patients, since it is associated with minimal hemodynamic depression.

MUSCLE RELAXANTS

Skeletal muscle relaxants have long been an element in the armamentarium of a balanced anesthesia induction sequence. Griffith and Johnson described the use of curare in general anesthesia for muscle relaxation[94]. Scurr emphasized the short-acting nature of succinyl-choline predicting success as a muscle relaxant[95]. Forbes and colleagues reported the ability of pancuronium, a longer-acting agent, to decrease the subsequent anesthetic requirement[96].

Classification of neuromuscular blocking agents (NMBAs) proceeds according to mechanism of action and chemical structure (Table 7). The depolarizing agents are short-acting linear quaternary amine (NCH_3^+) compounds such as succinylcholine. The non-depolarizing agents are longer-acting bulky aromatic quaternary ammonium (NCH_4^+)

Table 6 Inhalational anesthetic agents

Agent	Analgesia	Cardiovascular	Pulmonary	Neurological	GI	Renal	Elimination
Desflurane (Suprane®)	+	tachycardia	laryngospasm apnea (pediatrics)	↑ICP		↓perfusion	respiratory
Enflurane (Ethrane®)	+	less dysrhythmia	↓ respiratory drive	tremor		↓	respiratory
Halothane (Fluothane®)	+/–	myocardial depression bradycardia SA/AV conduction	bronchodilatation	↑ICP ↓CVR ↓CBF	hepatitis	↓	respiratory
Isoflurane (Forane®)	+	coronary artery steal	↓respiratory drive	tremor		↓	respiratory
Nitrous oxide	++	sympathomimetic	↑PVR	thermoregulation		↓	respiratory

GI, gastrointestinal; ICP, intracranial pressure; CVR, cerebrovascular resistance, CBF, cerebral blood flow; SA/AV, sinoatrial/atrioventricular node; PVR, peripheral vascular resistance; +, effect; –, no effect; ↓, decrease; ↑, increase compounds such as curare, pancuronium, vecuronium or atracurium.

Normal neuromuscular transmission at the motor endplate begins with fast sodium channel influx at the nerve terminal and subsequent calcium influx, acetylcholine release from the presynaptic receptor and acetylcholine binding to the postsynaptic nicotinic cholinergic endplate receptor, the fast sodium influx resulting in postsynaptic depolarization, followed by potassium efflux resulting in postsynaptic calcium release and excitation–contraction coupling.

The mechanism of action of depolarizing compared to non-depolarizing agents includes non-competitive inhibition of the acetylcholine receptor in a somewhat biphasic response. Phase I or the 'depolarizing blockade' occurs when succinylcholine acts as a longer-acting acetylcholine analog causing persistent endplate depolarization, rendering it unresponsive to new stimulation, resulting in flaccid paralysis. The phase II or 'desensitization blockade' occurs when continued exposure to succinylcholine fails to prevent repolarization but the endplate remains relatively refractory to acetylcholine binding. Thus, the postsynaptic surface remains desensitized, as in non-depolarizing blockade, with a non-sustained response to tetanic stimulus with fatigue, and fade responses.

Characterization of the response of neuromuscular blocking agents allows differentiation of depolarizing or non-depolarizing action (Table 8). The depolarizing agents feature an 'all or none' response to train-of-four, tetanus

Table 7 Neuromuscular blocking agents

	Depolarizing	*Non-depolarizing*
	Non-competitive	**Competitive**
Ultrashort	quaternary amine decamethonium succinylcholine	quaternary ammonium
Short		mivacurium
Intermediate		rocuronium vecuronium (s) atracurium (b) cisatracurium (b)
Long		tubocurarine (b) metocurine (b) gallamine (b) pancuronium (s) doxacurium pipecuronium

(s), steroid; (b), benzylisquinolone

Table 8 Characterization of the response of neuromuscular blocking agents

	Depolarizing (all or none)	*Non-depolarizing* (decremental)
Twitch	decrease	decrease
Train-of-four (four-twitch stimulus)	–	fade
Train-of-four ratio	>0.7	<0.4
Tetanus	–	+
Post-tetanic potentiation	–	+
Fade	–	+
Fasciculation	+	–
Onset	rapid	slow
Recovery	rapid	slow

or fade stimulus. The non-depolarizing agents feature a 'decremental' response to these stimuli, as well as post-tetanic potentiation.

The facilitation and potentiation of neuromuscular blockade may be affected in the critically ill, resulting in a delayed onset, but prolonged duration, of effect due to temperature, ionic instability and interaction with other pharmacological agents[97,98] (Table 9).

Depolarizing neuromuscular blocking agents

Discussion of depolarizing NMBAs centers on the only available induction agent succinylcholine. This non-competitive agent is administered in a 1.5-mg/kg intravenous dose and a 2–4.0-mg/kg intramuscular dose. The intravenous dose is increased to 2.0 mg/kg if a non-depolarizing agent is preadministered to prevent muscle fasciculation. The drug has the shortest (45–60 s) onset of action, along with a brief duration (5–15 min) of effect after hematological degradation by pseudocholinesterase and renal elimination. Adverse reactions include arrythmia due to muscarinic and nicotinic stimulation, hyperkalemia in those predisposed by burns, crush or denervation injury, and increased intraocular, gastric and intracranial pressure[93].

There are additional drug effects to consider, such as tachyphylaxis with the

Table 9 Potentiation of neuromuscular blockade. From references 97 and 98

Environmental
   Hypothermia
Anesthetics
   Inhalation
Metabolic
   Respiratory acidosis, metabolic alkalosis
Electrolyte
   Increased magnesium and lithium, decreased
      potassium
Antibiotics
   Aminoglycosides, ureidopenicillins, peptides,
      tetracycline
Antiarrhythmics
   Lidocaine, procainamide
Antihypertensive
   Calcium channel antagonist, trimethaphan

progressive nature of phase I depolarizing blockade at low doses (2–3 mg/kg) of succinylcholine to phase II non-depolarizing blockade at higher doses (5–6 mg/kg). The incidence of plasma cholinesterase deficiency is rare – heterozygous 1 in 25, homozygous 1 in 2800 – but failed hydrolysis to succinylmonocholine may prolong block. An even rarer complication is malignant hyperthermia, occurring in 1 in 50 000 anesthetics, which can be associated with succinylcholine administration.

Thus, the paradox is that succinylcholine, the most rapid acting and clinically useful NMBA has the most significant and diverse adverse effect profile. Review of clinical experience allows delineation of efficacy, as well as hierarchy of contraindications.

The utility of rapid-sequence intubation in the urgent setting has been reported by Talucci and co-workers to occur in 81% of 320 cases intubated orally from a retrospective evaluation of 335 patients[99]. Cicala and Westbrook compared relaxant induction sequences of *d*-tubocurarine (3 mg intravenously), thiopental (3–5 mg/kg), succinylcholine (1.5 mg/kg) and vecuronium (0.01 mg/kg + 0.14 mg/kg), thiopental (3–5 mg/kg) and fentanyl (3 μg/kg)[100]. Where intubating conditions were obtained in succinylcholine-treated patients more commonly than in vecuronium-treated cases (32 vs. 24 of 50), with quicker onset (69 vs. 174 s) and resolution (5.4 vs. 41 min) with succinylcholine.

The use of a defasciculating dose of NMBA, where a 10% normal dose of non-depolarizing agent is administered prior to an induction dose of a depolarizing agent, may potentially decrease muscle fasciculation and contraction. However, each of these potential side-effects of succinylcholine should be examined critically.

Gastric reflux was examined by Gorback and Graubert in 40 patients, of whom half were prone to reflux by history[101]. There was a decrease in esophageal pH in five of 20 reflux and none of 20 normal patients with no change noted with either succinylcholine induction or defasciculation. However, Salem and co-workers evaluated 30 pediatric patients demonstrating an increase in intragastric pressor of $\geq 4\,cmH_2O$ in five of 30 patients (16.6%), which was decreased with administration of a defasciculation agent[102].

Postoperative myalgias were evaluated by Sosis and associates: a defasciculating agent – atracurium (0.025 mg/kg), d-tubocurarine (0.05 mg/kg) or placebo – was administered in conjunction with succinylcholine[103]. Fasciculation was decreased in those who received d-tubocurarine (12%), compared to atracurium (46%) or placebo (79%), while the incidence of postoperative myalgia was decreased with atracurium (15%), d-tubocurarine (41%) and placebo (57%). Thus, d-tubocurarine is the better defasciculant, but atracurium results in less postinduction pain.

Intraocular pressure increase has been noted with depolarizing agents. Joshi and Bruce evaluated a low-dose (0.5 mg/kg) and high-dose (1.0 mg/kg) succinylcholine induction sequence and demonstrated that thiopental lowered the intraocular pressure, the low-dose succinylcholine regimen returned it to baseline, while the high-dose regimen increased the intraocular pressure[104]. In addition, they noted that the response in unprepared intubation was significantly greater than after administration of succinylcholine alone. Libonati and co-workers evaluated 100 pediatric open-eye repair patients pretreated with curare (3–6 mg), thiopental (150–250 mg) and succinylcholine (60–160 mg) with all cases (63 of 63) protected from vitreous extrusion[105].

Pediatric patients may be especially sensitive to succinylcholine-induced adverse effects. Pediatric patients induced with thiopental and succinylcholine demonstrated a 0.23-mmol/l potassium increase[106]. Van Der Spek and colleagues compared succinylcholine with vecuronium or pancuronium, resulting in a decrease in mean mouth opening, and increased jaw stiffness due to 'masseter spasm'[107].

An important consideration in the emergency induction sequence involves those with increased intracranial pressure. Minton and associates noted a 24% increase in intracranial pressure from 15.2 ± 1.3 to 20.1 ± 2.0 mmHg with five of 15 (33%) having a clinically significant (≥ 9 mmHg) increase[108]. They concluded that succinylcholine increased intracranial

pressure in the reduced intracranial compliance scenario, which was blunted only by a full relaxing dose (0.14 mm/kg) rather than a defasciculating dose (0.01 mg/kg) of vecuronium.

However, Kovarik and associates reported that succinylcholine (1 mg/kg) administered to ten mechanically ventilated patients with median Glasgow Coma Score of 6 (range 3–10) compared to saline placebo resulted in no appreciable change in intracranial pressure, cerebral perfusion pressure, the electroencephalogram (EEG), mean arterial pressure or mean middle cerebral artery (MCA) velocity[109].

Succinylcholine is the standard NMBA used in the emergency induction sequence providing rapid onset and rapid return of function, while side-effects are largely modified by the addition of a non-depolarizing defasciculating agent, except for hyperkalemia found in those with chronic denervation syndromes or disuse atrophy. The hierarchy of relative contraindications, including intracranial pressure elevation, gastric reflux and intraocular pressure elevation, need to be considered on a case-by-case basis.

Non-depolarizing neuromuscular blocking agents

Issues particular to the non-depolarizing NMBA class include a delayed decremental onset of action. There are two strategies suggested to compensate for the failure of the non-depolarizing agents to cause complete relaxation analogous to the 'all or none' loss of protectives associated with the depolarizing agents. The 'priming dose' concept suggests that the administration of a relaxant dose of 10% followed by a dose of 90% results in a decreased time until onset of the drug effect, without prolonging the duration of action. The 'slug dose' of 2–3 times the normal dose is associated with a decreased onset, but also a prolonged duration of effect.

Kunjappan and co-workers compared vecuronium administered in a 'back loaded' priming strategy (10 μg/kg prime and 130 μg, 140 μg/kg bolus), with succinylcholine

1.5 mg/kg, resulting in longer mean intubation times[110]. However, if the vecuronium primary dose was increased to 15 μg/kg and the bolus decreased to 100 μg/kg, this 'front loaded' strategy approximated the intubating conditions of succinylcholine administration. Huemer and associates compared priming dose variation (10, 15, 20 μg/kg) followed in 6 min by bolus vecuronium administration, and observed no difference in time to intubating conditions[111].

Davison and Holland, in a comparison of non-depolarizing agents, demonstrated a mean intubation time of 75 s for succinylcholine, 149 s for vecuronium and 164 s for atracurium, measured as 80–90% twitch depression[112]. Even with a primary strategy, neither non-depolarizing agent approached the effectiveness of succinylcholine.

Silverman and co-workers commented on the extensive dosing variability of the non-depolarizing agent at a factor of 1–6 times the median effective dose (ED_{50})[113]. Their study of 75 ASA I/II patients compared vecuronium with succinylcholine (1.5 mg/kg) and found a 73% range of response, but an onset of action measured as time to 95% twitch height depression decreased from 120 to 95 s with a priming dose. Mortier and colleagues evaluated an atracurium priming strategy (100 + 300 μg/kg) compared to vecuronium (20 + 60 μg/kg) in 20 elective gynecological patients, and noted no difference in speed of onset measured as T190 s (23.5% vs. 14.6%) or duration measured as T150 s (41.3% vs. 34.2%)[114].

Information concerning the accelerated bolus strategy can be extrapolated from the dose range study of vecuronium by Yamada and Takino. The optimal dose was 0.15 mg/kg, which was associated with a time of onset measured as 90% relaxation at 135 s with recovery of 25% of strength occurring at 63 min, compared to 0.10 to 0.20 mg/kg[115].

There are many commonly available non-depolarizing agents currently used, most of moderate or prolonged action (Table 10)[116–119]. There are several newer agents that claim 'closely' to approximate the characteristics of succinylcholine that need to be examined.

d-Tubocurarine was the first non-depolarizing agent used for muscle relaxation. The dose is 0.03 mg/kg intravenously for defasciculation or 0.5 mg/kg for intubation with the onset of action within 3 min and a 30-min duration of effect. The drug undergoes renal and biliary excretion causing competitive blockade of the acetylcholine receptor through a non-depolarizing mechanism. This agent has significant side-effects, including histamine-mediated vasodilatation, ganglionic blockade and direct myocardial depression.

Clinical use of d-tubocurarine as a single agent is encountered only rarely, owing to significant adverse cardiovascular effects such as hypotension. Goudsouzian and colleagues compared d-tubocurarine (0.8 mg/kg) and pancuronium (0.13 mg/kg) in 27 pediatric patients, and demonstrated equivalent intubating conditions, including time to maximal effect, muscle relaxation and recovery time[120]. This cardiovascular effect potentiates the arterial hypotensive effect of thiopental, as well as acting as a direct myocardial depressant, but may prevent adrenergic-mediated dysrhythmia due to calcium antagonism[121].

The most commonly administered non-depolarizing agent is vecuronium bromide. The dose for defasciculation is 0.01 mg/kg and for relaxation is 0.1 mg/kg. The advantage of this drug is the rapid onset within 2–4 min with a moderate 20–30-min duration of effect, and it is relatively free of vagolytic activity or histamine release.

Vecuronium was compared with succinylcholine in an early study by Williams and co-workers, who concluded that acceptable intubating conditions were obtained in only 30% of 40 patients. They stated that 'the action is too slow for rapid intubation'[122]. Complete relaxation was obtained in 100% of the succinylcholine (1 mg/kg) patients, and in 7–13% of the vecuronium (50–90 μg/kg) patients. Forstmann and Schuh compared vecuronium (0.10 mg/kg) and atracurium (0.5 mg/kg) with succinylcholine (1.0 mg/kg) in 205 patients, and again noted a superior response (98% blockade) with succinylcholine, while vecuronium (85%) and atracurium (86%) were equivalent[123].

Table 10 Neuromuscular blocking agents. From references 116–119

Classification	Structure	Type	Dose (mg/kg)	Onset (min)	Duration (min)	Infusion (μg/kg per min)	Elimination (% elimination)	HR (%)	BP (%)	Histamine	Side-effects
Depolarizing											
Succinylcholine	ester	ultrashort	1–2	1	5–10	50	Pseudocholinesterase	–	–	–	inc. K, ICP, IOP, malignant hypothermia
Non-depolarizing											
Mivacurium	bq	short	0.1	2–4	20	10	renal, hepatic	+10	–20	+	hypotension
Rocuronium	s mono	short	0.5	1.5	30		hepatic	–	–	–	–
Vecuronium	s mono	moderate	0.1	3–5	20–45	70	biliary (40%) renal (20%)	–	–	–	–
Atracurium	bq	moderate	0.5	3–5	20–45		autolysis	+15	–20	+	hypotension
Cisatracurium	bq	moderate	0.2	2–3	30		autolysis	–	–	–	–
d-Tubocurarine	bq	long	0.5	3–5	30	400	renal (50%) hepatic (50%)	+25	–25	++	hypotension
Pancuronium	s bi	long	0.06	3–5	60–90	25	biliary (30%) renal (20%)	+20	–	–	vagolytic
Pipecuronium	s	ultralong	0.04	3–6	40–110		renal	–	–	–	–
Doxacurium	bq	ultralong	0.04	3.5–10	77–164		renal	–	–	–	–

HR, heart rate; BP, blood pressure; K, potassium; ICP, intracranial pressure; IOP, intraocular pressure; s, steroidal analog; mono, monoquaternary; bi, biquaternary; bq, benzylisoquinolinium

It is crucial to note that there appears to be significant variability in the action of non-depolarizing NMBAs. The onset of action of vecuronium may range from 2.04 to 2.97 min with excellent intubating conditions obtained in 50–90% of cases[124]. Silverman and associates found 75% variance in the onset of 95% twitch height depression for 75 patients receiving 1.5–6 times the dose estimated to achieve the effective dose in 95% (ED_{95}), but with five of 16 patients requiring >120 s for relaxation[113].

An increased dosing strategy of 0.3 mg/kg of vecuronium administered as a single dose still required 140 s to the onset of intubating conditions, not much decreased from standard dosing[125]. Interestingly, a divided priming strategy (0.015, 0.285 mg/kg) resulted in a decreased time (80 s) to adequate intubating conditions. Thus, increasing the administered dose measured as 0.5–1.5 × ED_{95} results in a linear increase in duration of action, but does not affect time to onset[126].

Clinical comparison of vecuronium (0.3 mg/kg) and succinylcholine (1.0 mg/kg) found that, 60 s after administration, good intubating conditions were obtained in 96% of both groups[127]. The suggestion is that the efficacy of vecuronium is equivalent to succinylcholine only at a higher dose, and benefits may be offset by extended duration of action, which is problematic in an emergency failed airway.

Atracurium besylate is administered in a dose of 0.5 (0.3–0.6) mg/kg with moderate onset of action within 2–4 min and a 30–45-min duration of effect. The drug's advantages include its non-enzymatic mode of degradation, the 'Hoffman' elimination process and ester hydrolysis, while the disadvantages include histamine release[118].

The primary principle has also been described for the administration of atracurium. Gergis and associates compared a primary dosing strategy for atracurium (0.08, 0.42 mg/kg), standard dose (0.5 mg/kg) atracurium and succinylcholine (1.0 mg/kg), and noted good relaxation in 90–100% of patients who were improved with the divided dose strategy[128]. Studies comparing atracurium and succinylcholine suggest equivalent intubation

conditions by 2 min with the benefit of cardiovascular stability[129]. However, Famewo's evaluation of 60 patients suggested that atracurium in a 0.5–0.7-mg/kg dose range required twice the time for onset (120 vs. 60 s) compared to succinylcholine[130].

Atracurium is most often recommended for use in those with renal failure or other elimination difficulties. Hunter and co-workers utilized this agent in 26 anephric patients at a 0–3-mg/kg induction and 2–3-mg/kg maintenance dose, demonstrating no accumulation or adverse cardiovascular effects compared to those with normal renal function[131]. This is significant in that histamine release is cited as an adverse effect of atracurium.

Another consideration may be the association with an increased likelihood of seizure activity. NMBAs may cause excitatory phenomena involving the activation of cerebral acetylcholine or glutamate receptors, mediated by increased calcium influx in postsynaptic neurons often associated with pancuronium and vecuronium administration[132]. D,L-laudanosine, an atracurium metabolite, has been identified with an inhibitory effect directed to the low-infinity γ-aminobutyric acid (GABA) receptors increasing seizure activity, as well as to opioid binding sites[133].

There has been a resurgence of interest concerning pancuronium, owing to economic considerations. Pancuronium bromide is administered in a 0.1-mg/kg dose with onset within 2–4 min. This is a long-acting drug (3–60 min) with a side-effect profile including a vagolytic and sympathomimetic influence causing tachycardia or hypertension.

The use of pancuronium was described by Roizen and Feeley in 1978, when succinylcholine was contraindicated, to facilitate intubation and minimize bronchospasm, muscle spasm associated with tetanus, tremor or shivering[134]. This agent may be suitable for induction in cases when prolonged paralysis is acceptable.

The onset of action may be decreased by a priming strategy. Mehta and colleagues compared a pancuronium priming dose (0.015 mg/kg), followed by pancuronium (0.08 mg/kg) or atracurium (0.4 mg/kg), with good intubating conditions by 60 s in 100% of pancuronium cases and 83% of atracurium cases[135]. This drug is probably not suited to emergency intubation conditions. Monitoring documented both hypertension, with 11–15% increase in blood pressure and 30–39% increase in heart rate, and prolonged duration of action compared to vecuronium (37–25 min)[136].

Schaer and co-workers compared pancuronium (0.08–0.11 mg/kg), vecuronium (0.07–0.10 mg/kg) and atracurium (0.35–0.5 mg/kg), and demonstrated equivalent time of onset, with intubating conditions at 2 min for high-dose and 3 min for low-dose therapy, but prolonged recovery time (two-fold increase) for pancuronium compared to the other agents[117]. Thus, the clinical evaluation of pancuronium (0.08–0.1 mg/kg) and atracurium (0.6–0.8 mg/kg) in 96 patients by Twohig and colleagues suggests that neither drug was effective before 60 s, with an 11% failure rate and atracurium performing slightly better[137]. Again, as for atracurium, the side-effect profile combined with a delayed onset and prolonged duration of action makes pancuronium an unlikely choice for an emergency induction sequence.

Consideration of the newer class of non-depolarizing muscle relaxants is warranted. The addition of extended duration agents such as doxacurium and pipecuronium has little clinical relevance in the emergency intubation scenario.

Mivacurium chloride was the first of a new class of shorter-acting agents based, like atracurium, on the benzylisoquinolinium diester structure. This drug is administered in a 0.1–0.2-mg/kg intubating dose providing $2 \times ED_{95}$ for a 15–20-min duration followed by rapid plasma cholinesterase elimination[138].

The benefits of the drug are the avoidance of cumulative neuromuscular blockade or 'recurarization' typical of longer-acting agents. Disadvantages include the same prolonged paralysis associated with other agents in the homozygous atypical plasma cholinesterase condition along with cardiovascular instability associated with histamine release[138].

Dose range evaluation comparing 0.03–0.30 mg/kg of mivacurium determined the

ED_{95} to be 0.08 mg/kg. Routine indications warranted a 0.10-mg/kg dose with onset in 3.8 min and recovery within 24 min, while for rapid induction, sequences using the augmented dose (0.25 mg/kg) with significant adjunct anesthesia including nitrous oxide, narcotic and thiopental decreased the onset time to 2.3 min and the duration of effect to 30 min[139].

Mivacurium has been compared with standard intubation sequences containing either succinylcholine or vecuronium. Goldberg and associates compared mivacurium (0.2–0.25 mg/kg) at $3 \times ED_{95}$ and succinylcholine (1.0 mg/kg), demonstrating equivalent intubating conditions at 2 min for mivacurium and 1 min for succinylcholine[140]. The duration of effect was half as long for succinylcholine (6 min) compared to mivacurium (13 min). Mangat and co-workers performed a similar comparison in children, and demonstrated a two-fold increase in time until onset of block for mivacurium (143 s) compared to succinylcholine (56 s)[141].

The major difficulty with mivacurium is that the time of onset and duration of effect, although decreased compared to the moderate-duration agents vecuronium and atracurium, do not approach the conditions achieved with succinylcholine, the optimal 'ultrashort' NMBA for emergency induction sequences.

Mivacurium has also been compared with the newer NMBAs. The time until relaxation after administration of the $2 \times ED_{90}$ dose of mivacurium was greater (229 s) than in either vecuronium (192 s) or rocuronium (172 s); however, the duration of action was shortest with mivacurium (13, 33, 28 min)[142].

Rocuronium bromide may be the first 'rapid onset' non-depolarizing agent. Rocuronium is administered in a 0.6-mg/kg dose with onset in 1–2 min and an average 46-min duration of effect. The drug is degraded predominantly by the liver, but may accumulate in those patients with renal failure. The presence of hepatic dysfunction results in a 25% increase in volume of distribution from 5.96 to 7.87 l with a corresponding 32% prolongation of elimination half-life from 75 to 111 min[143]. Khuenl-Brady and associates evaluated the use of rocuronium in those with chronic renal failure and demonstrated equivalent induced and spontaneous recovery indices, suggesting absence of cumulative block[144].

The intubating conditions achieved with rocuronium (0.6 mg/kg) compared to succinylcholine found both acceptable at 60–90 s[145]. Interestingly, however, there was a discrepancy between the objective adductor pollicis strength measurement compared to the subjective ease of laryngoscopy measure. Clinical evaluation exploring variable dose regimens (0.6–0.9 mg/kg) and onset times (45, 60 s) suggested optimal intubation time in the latter, but found no effect of dosage increase[146]. Dubois and co-workers used a double-blinded design comparing rocuronium (0.6 mg/kg) to succinylcholine (1 mg/kg) with onset times of 130 and 74 s, respectively, and no significant cardiovascular effects[147].

Another 'blinded' clinical comparison of rocuronium and succinylcholine found equivalent intubation conditions at 60 s, although time to spontaneous recovery (25–75%) was shorter for succinylcholine (2.2 vs. 7.8 min)[148]. Magorian and colleagues compared rocuronium (0.6–1.2 mg/kg), vecuronium (0.1 mg/kg) and succinylcholine (1.0 mg/kg), and demonstrated equivalent onset times for higher-dose rocuronium (0.9 mg/kg) and succinylcholine (55, 50 s), whereas vecuronium required 144 s[149].

An issue in the use of both rocuronium and mivacurium is that, to optimize intubating conditions, a balanced induction sequence involving multiple agents is required, decreasing utility in the emergency situation. Crul and co-workers compared rocuronium and succinylcholine accompanied by alfentanil (20 μg/kg) and propofol (2–2.5 mg/kg), with excellent intubating conditions obtained in the rocuronium group, for 55% of patients receiving the 0.6-mg/kg dose and 90% of those receiving the 0.9-mg/kg dose, at 45–60 s[150]. Rapid-sequence comparison of intubating conditions after rocuronium (0.6 mg/kg) and succinylcholine (1.5 mg/kg) along with thiopental was performed. The investigators noted that all patients could be intubated within 60 s[151]. Interestingly, a 0.04-mg/kg priming dose of rocuronium did not hasten successful intubation.

A reasonable conclusion is that this drug most closely approximates the succinylcholine efficacy in the emergency induction, but owing to its variability of onset and longer duration of action, succinylcholine remains the agent of choice.

Another recently released agent is cisatracurium besylate, with claims of the cardiovascular stability of vecuronium, accompanied by the disintegration mode of elimination of atracurium. The recommended intubating dose is 0.2 mg/kg which is $4 \times ED_{95}$ establishing acceptable conditions within 90 s with fentanyl, midazolam and propofol as adjuncts to induction.

This drug undergoes 'Hofmann elimination', as does atracurium to laudanosine and a monoquaternary alcohol with a half-life of 29.2 ± 3.8 min[152]. Cisatracurium is safe for use in those with hepatic and renal dysfunction, although neurological issues concerning the effect of laudanosine on seizure threshold should be considered.

Cardiovascular effects due to histamine release and ganglionic blockade are greater for steroid analogs than for benzylisoquinolinium compounds (atracurium, mivacurium), and within the steroid group greater for monoquaternary (d-tubocurarine, vecuronium) than bisquaternary (pancuronium) drugs. Konstadt and co-workers compared cisatracurium (0.10 mg/kg) and vecuronium (0.10 mg/kg) in 70 elective myocardial revascularization patients for postintubation relaxation and found no adverse hemodynamic effect for either agent[153]. Prielipp and colleagues reported more prolonged blockade with vecuronium than cisatracurium after continuous infusion therapy in 58 ventilated critically ill patients in the intensive care unit[154].

Rapacuronium is a non-depolarizing NMBA with a rapid intubation indication for short surgical procedures and a dose range of 1.5 mg/kg for adults, 2 mg/kg for pediatric patients and 2.5 mg/kg for cesarean section[155]. The drug has an elimination half-life ($t_{1/2}$) of 141 min with a side-effect profile that includes hypotension (5%) and bronchospasm (3.2%).

However, this drug has been substituted as a succinylcholine alternative with a mean onset of action of 90 s and a mean blockade duration of 15 (6–30) min if a depolarizing agent is undesirable.

Clinical trials suggest that rapacuronium (1.5 mg/kg) performs favorably compared to decreased succinylcholine (1 mg/kg) or mivacurium (0.25 mg/kg to 0.15 mg/kg followed in 30 s by 0.10 mg/kg), with a mean onset of action and duration of action of 98 s and 15 min, 6 min and 9 min, and 127 s and 21 min, respectively[156]. The authors also found acceptable intubating conditions with a 1.5 mg/kg rapacuronium and 1 mg/kg succinylcholine dose at 50 s with acceptable intubating conditions in 85–90% and 89–97% of patients, respectively.

It appears that, of the newest class of NMBAs, rapacuronium, rocuronium or mivacurium is best suited for emergency induction sequences, although still not approved by the Food and Drug Administration (FDA). However, there is no non-depolarizing agent that is as effective as succinylcholine for this indication. Moreover, rapacuronium may be associated with occasional adverse side-effects that may prohibit further development.

Reversal of neuromuscular blockade

The autonomic nervous system (ANS) consists of the sympathetic nervous system, utilizing norepinephrine and interacting with α, β and dopaminergic receptors; and the parasympathetic nervous system, mediated by acetylcholine interacting with nicotinic receptors at the neuromuscular junction and muscarinic receptors at postganglionic nerve terminals.

The reversal of neuromuscular blockade may be attempted in the proper clinical setting. The anticholinesterase inhibitor (ACE-I) agents bind to acetylcholinesterase, preventing acetylcholine degradation, to increase motor endplate concentration of this neurotransmitter.

The tertiary compounds include pyridostigmine (15 mg/kg) administered in a 0.5–1.0-mg intravenous dose, but it is not used, owing to its CNS penetration and subsequent effects. The quaternary nitrogen compounds most commonly used include neostigmine (0.005–0.05 mg/kg) administered in a standard 2.5-mg (0.5–3.5) dose and pyridostigmine (0.02–0.2 mg/kg) administered in a 10–20-mg dose. Edrophonium (0.1–0.4 mg/kg) can be administered in a 7–10-mg dose but is not commonly used for this indication.

Donati and co-workers evaluated these three agents in 120 elective surgical cases with 90% recovery of first twitch height after pancuronium and d-tubocurarine relaxation[157]. The first twitch ED_{50} for neostigmine was 0.013–0.017, for pyridostigmine 0.085–0.11 and edrophonium 0.17–0.27, with neostigmine being the most potent agent, but some variability in effectiveness depending on the NMBA used.

The higher end of the dose range should be used in urgent cases of reversal. For routine reversal, however, doses used should be guided by train-of-four testing. Full return of motor function may require 5 min for neostigmine and 10 min for pyridostigmine, limiting their use in a difficult airway scenario.

An anticholinergic agent, such as atropine (0.02 mg/kg) administered in a 0.6-mg standard dose or glycopyrrolate (0.005 mg/kg) administered in a 0.4-mg dose is used in conjunction to offset the muscarinic effects of the ACE-I such as bradycardia or excess secretions. The timing of atropine premedication warrants administration prior to the ACE-I for best protection[158].

Reversal of paralysis is not a substitute for adequate airway control in the emergency setting, and some temporizing strategy is often necessary.

CLINICAL SCENARIOS

Emergency induction regimens using neuromuscular blockers need to be modified and adapted to individual clinical circumstances, patient stability and disease states (Figure 16).

Cardiac dysfunction

Cardiovascular dysfunction warrants caution to avoid significant hypotension and subsequent

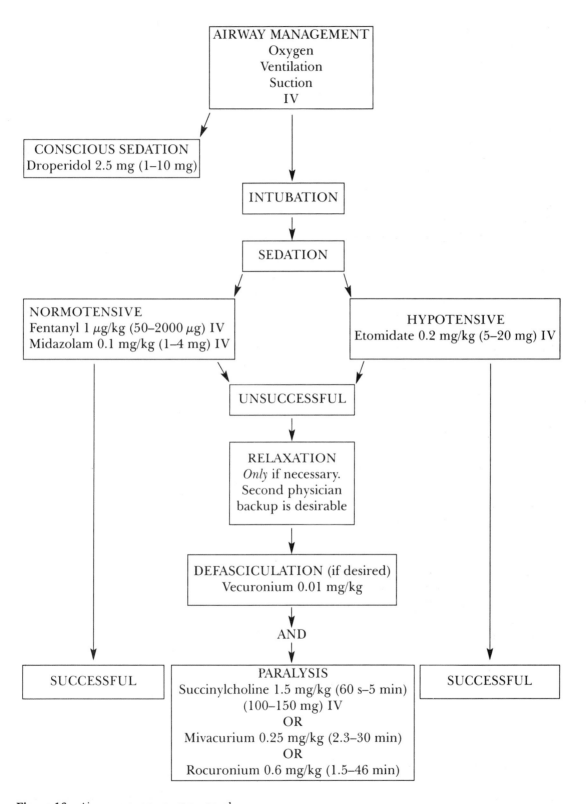

Figure 16 Airway management protocol

myocardial ischemia. Larach and colleagues evaluated 64 patients with valvular disease[159], citing specific concerns in patients with mitral stenosis and aortic stenosis not to decrease preload significantly during induction, while mitral and aortic regurgitation are better able to compensate[158]. There appear to be minimal hemodynamic effects with vecuronium, while atracurium creates a hyperdynamic state with increased cardiac index (CI) and decreased systemic vascular resistance index (SVRI), while pancuronium acts as a myocardial depressant decreasing CI and increasing SVRI[159].

Sethna and co-workers compared the cardiovascular effects of muscle relaxants, and found that pancuronium was associated with significant tachycardia (+23 vs. 2% heart rate), atracurium associated with decrease in peripheral tone (–18 vs. 1% SVRI), while vecuronium had relatively little effect[160]. Therefore, induction of patients at risk for ischemia requires preload maintenance, hemodynamically favorable sedation or analgesia – etomidate or fentanyl – and a relaxant associated with cardiovascular stability – succinylcholine or vecuronium.

Trauma

The trauma population poses a difficult intubation situation based on factors such as recent oral intake, anatomic difficulties, patient compliance and cervical spine positioning issues. Redan and associates evaluated 100 trauma patients, who underwent rapid sequence induction with vecuronium (59%) or succinylcholine (41%) with a 3% failure rate requiring cricothyroidotomy[161]. The incidence of patients requiring endotracheal intubation after presenting to a level I trauma center was 18.6% from the evaluation of Talucci and colleagues of 1798 consecutive patients[99]. Rapid-sequence induction was used in 81% of patients with success in all cases without adverse hemodynamic sequelae (Figure 17).

Ligier and colleagues evaluated rapid-sequence induction in a group of 97 severely injured trauma patients, and reported that

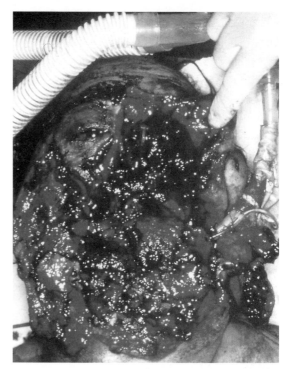

Figure 17 Catastrophic facial trauma

use of relaxants facilitated intubation (100%) with 92% on the first attempt compared to 61% in control patients[162]. Again, the failed intubation rate requiring cricothyroidotomy was 4%. This was similar to the aeromedical experience of Syverud and co-workers, using a succinylcholine regimen in 74 patients, yielding a 96% success rate with only 46% intubated on the first attempt and a 4% arrythmia rate[163].

Head injury

Head injury, which may be accompanied by an increase in intracranial pressure, is often problematic, since administering 'brain-protective' agents may adversely affect systemic perfusion. However, the most detrimental situation, manifested as a significant rise in intracranial pressure with subsequent decrease in cerebral perfusion pressure, occurs with underventilation and hypercarbia, as well as in difficult intubation with multiple laryngoscopy attempts[164,165].

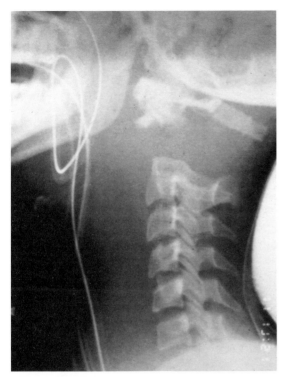

Figure 18   Presence of significant cervical trauma

Rapid-sequence induction should provide optimal cerebral protection from hypertensive rise, as well as relaxation to facilitate effective and atraumatic tracheal cannulation. Both diazepam and midazolam have been associated with success in blunting the intracranial pressure rise associated with intubation by as much as 35%[62,77]. This effect may be even greater for thiopental, while etomidate seems protective in this circumstance. The cerebral protection afforded by a narcotic analgesic, such as fentanyl, may be only moderate and indirect, but is reversible, allowing subsequent mental status examination.

The choice of NMBA again suggests that the major issue is adequate muscle relaxation, not the decision of whether a depolarizing or non-depolarizing agent is to be used. Minton and associates evaluated the intracranial pressure change associated with succinyl-choline administration and found a minimum increase of 2 mmHg with vecuronium pre-treatment to a maximum of 9 mmHg increase without defasciculation[108]. Rosa and co-workers evaluated vecuronium in 20 patients with intracranial tumor and found a 5% decrease in intracranial pressure accompanied by a 15% decrease in central venous pressure, with minimal adverse effect on cerebral or systemic hemodynamics[166]. Likewise, atracurium administered in a controlled ventilation model demonstrated no increase in intracranial pressure due to histamine release and subsequent compensatory cardiovascular response[167].

Therefore, the proper sequence should include an amnestic agent, preferably etomidate or fentanyl, accompanied by succinylcholine with a defasciculating dose of vecuronium.

Cervical injury

Another consideration is the presence of cervical injury or fracture, when considering intubation technique. Meschino and co-workers performed a retrospective case–control study in 454 patients, and demonstrated a 2.5% rate of new deficit, in either the awake intubation ($n = 165$) or the unintubated group ($n = 289$)[168]. Suderman and colleagues retrospectively examined 150 patients with known cervical injury; 33% demonstrated a preoperative single-level radiculopathy, with a 6.6% rate of difficult intubation requiring more than one attempt[169]. However, there were two patients (1.3%) with new defects, but these were not correlated with maneuver of induction, route of intubation or in-line stabilization technique (Figure 18).

Rhee and co-workers examined emergency intubation in 237 trauma patients, where cervical injury occurred in 9% of patients[170]. The direct oral intubation route was chosen in most patients and not a single case of new deficit was identified. Careful technique and in-line stabilization is essential to prevent further cervical damage.

Hauswald and colleagues performed a postmortem cinefluoroscopic study, demonstrating that the most significant amount of movement occurred with mask ventilation (2.93 mm) compared to any other aspect of intubation[171]. Majernick and associates examined specific aspects of intubation. They reported that only in-line stabilization decreased cervical movement, while blade design and a rigid cervical collar had no effect[172]. Aprahamian and co-workers used an experimental cervical spine model to delineate the greatest cervical displacement (5 mm), which occurred with the chin-lift, jaw-thrust airway maneuver or nasal intubation[173]. An additional observation was that the one-piece rigid collar prevented spinal movement, while the two-piece semirigid device was less helpful.

In-line stabilization was compared to traction in 17 blunt trauma arrest patients in which four had an unstable fracture, such as $C_{6,7}$ fracture–dislocation, hangman's fracture and atlanto-occipital dislocation, to demonstrate up to 7.75 mm of distraction and 4 mm of subluxation with applied axial traction[174]. Therefore, with experienced anesthesiologists providing in-line stabilization, the rate of new deficit can be minimized (0%) based on the retrospective survey of 81 patients by Scannell and colleagues[175]. This series had a 12% incidence of initial deficit, 47% unstable fracture, and 28% stable fracture.

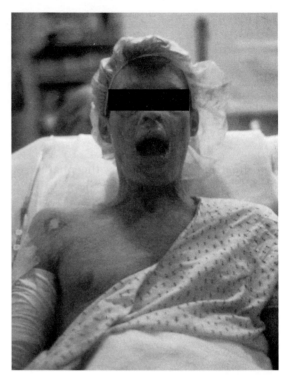

Figure 19 Burn patient with oropharyngeal scarring

Penetrating neck injury

The presence of penetrating neck injury is associated with a multiplicity of injuries, including vascular, tracheobronchial or pharyngoesophageal trauma. Eggen and Jorfen examined 114 patients retrospectively and, of this group, 23% were intubated as an emergency, 38% electively, and 39% were not intubated[176]. The crucial point was that adequate relaxation is essential for successful intubation, owing to the potential for vascular compromise and subsequent hemorrhage, hematoma and airway occlusion.

Burn or immobilization

There has been an extraordinary amount of discussion concerning the use of depolarizing vs. non-depolarizing agents in light of potential adverse effects. The use of succinylcholine in burn patients was evaluated by Schaner and associates in a canine model; they reported that there was dose-related hyperkalemia for succinylcholine doses of 0.7 mg/kg (5.44 ± 0.90 mmol K+) and 1.4 mg/kg (5.8 ± 1.14 mmol K+)[177]. Further, the rise in potassium was not extensive (1.23–1.73 mmol) and occurred late (20–30 days) in the burn course, with only extensive (>50%) burn, and the electrocardiogram was found to be an insensitive measure of potassium level. Therefore, succinylcholine is probably not harmful when administered in the patient with an acute burn, although there is no risk of this complication with a non-depolarizing agent in the acute injury phase.

However, there is a significant risk of hyperkalemia in those patients who are immobilized and are administered succinylcholine. Gronert and Theye studied a canine gastrocnemius muscle preparation and noted a 5 mmol/min per 100 g tissue flux in normal models, 20 mmol in immobilized preparations,

100 mmol in paraplegic and 130 mmol in denervated muscle preparations[178]. This acetylcholine receptor down-regulation phenomenon results in increased sensitivity, and consequently succinylcholine should be avoided in those who are immobilized.

Liver disease

The final issue is to address the pharmaco-kinetic profile of the critically ill patient best typified by those with cirrhosis. Van Beem and colleagues compared the metabolism of etomidate in five cirrhotic patients to report normal clearance rates, but prolonged elimination half-life based on a two-fold increase of volume of distribution[179], Therefore, in the critically ill patient, the initial bolus dose may need to be increased, while subsequent infusion therapy is curtailed, to obtain adequate intubating conditions without prolonged activity.

CONCLUSION

The successful endotracheal intubation requires adequate assessment, preparation and knowledge of indications for the procedure. The experienced practitioner should be familiar with a wide variety of anesthesia induction agents and neuromuscular blocking drugs.

The standard training pathway begins with awake intubation, progressing to sedation and rapid sequence induction strategies. It is essential to be aware of individual disease processes and their potential modification of pharmacological regimens used for endotracheal intubation.

References

1. MacEwen W. Clinical observations on the introduction of tracheal tubes by the mouth instead of performing tracheotomy or laryngotomy. *Br Med J* 1880;2:122–4

2. Kirstein A. Autoscopie des larynx und der trachea Berliner klin. *Wehnschrift* 1895;32:476–8

3. Jackson C. The technique of insertion of intratracheal insufflation tubes. *Surg Gynecol Obstet* 1913;17:507–9

4. Guedel AS, Waters RM. A new intratracheal catheter. *Anesth Analg* 1928;7:238–9

5. Flagg PJ. Introduction. In Flagg PJ, ed. *The Art of Anaesthesia*. Philadelphia and London: JB Lippincott, 1916:1–9

6. Guedel AE. Third stage ether anesthesia. *Natl Anesth Res Soc Bull* 1920;3:1–4

7. Lundy JS. Balanced anesthesia. *Minn Med* 1926;9:399–404

8. Knight RG, Castro T, Rastrelli AJ, Maschke S, Scavone JA. Arterial blood pressure and heart rate response to lighted stylet or direct laryngoscopy for endotracheal intubation. *Anesthesiology* 1988;69:269–72

9. Hickey S, Cameron AE, Asbury AJ, Murray GD. Timing of peak pressor response following endotracheal intubation. *Acta Anaesthesiol Scand* 1992;36:21–4

10. Bruder N, Ortega D, Granthil C. Consequences and prevention methods of hemodynamic changes during laryngoscopy and intratracheal intubation [French]. *Ann Fr Anesth Reanim* 1992;11:57–71

11. Pathak D, Slater RM, Ping SS, From RP. Effects of alfentanil and lidocaine on the hemodynamic responses to laryngoscopy and tracheal intubation. *J Clin Anesth* 1990;2:81–5

12. Stoelting RK, Peterson C. Circulatory changes during anesthetic induction: impact of d-tubocurarine pretreatment, thiamylal, succinylcholine, laryngoscopy, and tracheal lidocaine. *Anesth Analg* 1976;55:77–81

13. Hassan HG, el-Sharkawy TY, Renck H, Mansour G, Fouda A. Hemodynamic and catecholamine responses to laryngoscopy with vs. without endotracheal intubation. *Acta Anaesthesiol Scand* 1991;35:442–7

14. Stewart RD, Paris P, Pelton GH, Garretson D. Effect of varied training techniques on field endotracheal intubation success rates. *Ann Emerg Med* 1984;13:1032–6

15. O'Flaherty D, Adams AP. Endotracheal intubation skills of medical students. *J R Soc Med* 1992;85:603–4

16. Goldberg JS, Bernard AC, Marks RJ, Sladen RN. Simulation technique for difficult intubation: teaching tool or new hazard? *J Clin Anesth* 1990;2:21–6

17. Koller C. Historical notes on the beginning of local anesthesia. *J Am Med Assoc* 1928;90:1742–3

18. Knoefel PK, Herwick RP, Loevenhart AS. The prevention of acute intoxication from local anesthetics. *J Pharmacol Exp Ther* 1930;39:397–411

19. Magill IW. Endotracheal anaesthesia. *Proc R Soc Med* 1928;22:83

20. Gallager JV, Vance MV, Beechler C. Difficult nasotracheal intubation: a previously unreported anatomical cause. *Ann Emerg Med* 1985;14:258–60

21. Hartigan ML, Cleary JL, Schaffer DW. A comparison of pretreatment regimens for minimizing the hemodynamic response to blind nasotracheal intubation. *Can Anaesth Soc J* 1984;31:497–502

22. Dronen SC, Merigian KS, Hedges JR, Borron SW. A comparison of blind nasotracheal and succinylcholine-assisted intubation in the poisoned patient. *Ann Emerg Med* 1987;16:650–2

23. Fassolt A. Blind nasotracheal intubation in the muscle-relaxed patient [German]. *Anaesthetist* 1986;35:504–8

24. Thomas JL. Awake intubation indications, techniques and review of 25 patients. *Anaesthesia* 1969;24:28–35

25. Lee LS, Chau SW, Yu KL, *et al.* Clinical study of awake fiberoptic nasotracheal intubation for difficult opening mouth patients [Chinese]. *Ma Tsui Hsueh Tsa Chi* 1990;28:343–9

26. Redden RL, Biery KA, Campbell RL. Arterial oxygen desaturation during awake endotracheal intubation. *Anesth Prog* 1990;37:201–4

27. Hawkyard SJ, Morrison A, Doyle LA, Croton RS, Wake PN. Attenuating the hypertensive response to laryngoscopy and endotracheal intubation using awake fiberoptic intubation. *Acta Anaesthesiol Scand* 1992;36:1–4

28. Curran J, Hamilton C, Taylor T. Topical analgesia before tracheal intubation. *Anaesthesia* 1975;30:765–8

29. Stoelting RK. Circulatory changes during direct laryngoscopy and tracheal intubation: influence of duration of laryngoscopy with or without prior lidocaine. *Anesthesiology* 1975;17:43–4

30. Derbyshire DR, Smith G, Achola KJ. Effect of topical lignocaine on the sympathoadrenal responses to tracheal intubation. *Br J Anaesth* 1987;59:300–4

31. Hamill JF, Bedford RF, Weaver DC, Colohan AR. Lidocaine before endotracheal intubation: intravenous or laryngotracheal? *Anesthesiology* 1981;55:578–81

32. Denlinger JK, Ellison N, Ominsky AJ. Effects of intratracheal lidocaine on circulatory responses to tracheal intubation. *Anesthesiology* 1974;41:409–12

33. Chraemmer-Jorgensen B, Hoilund-Carlsen PF, Marving J, Christensen V. Lack of effect of intravenous lidocaine on hemodynamic responses to rapid sequence induction of general anesthesia: a double-blind controlled clinical trial. *Anesth Analg* 1986;65:1037–41

34. Abou-Madi M, Keszler H, Yacoub O. A method for prevention of cardiovascular reactions to laryngoscopy and intubation. *Can Anaesth Soc J* 1975;22:316–29

35. Boster SR, Danzl DF, Madden RJ, Jarboe CH. Translaryngeal absorption of lidocaine. *Ann Emerg Med* 1982;11:461–5

36. Mateer JR, Olson DW, Stueven HA, Aufderheide TP. Continuous pulse oximetry during emergency endotracheal intubation. *Ann Emerg Med* 1993;22:675–9

37. Gambee AM, Hertzka RE, Fisher DM. Preoxygenation techniques: comparison of three minutes and four breaths. *Anesth Analg* 1987;66:468–70

38. Sellick BA. Cricoid pressure to control regurgitation of stomach contents during induction of anesthesia. *Lancet* 1961;2:404–6

39. Petito SP, Russell WJ. The prevention of gastric inflation – a neglected benefit of cricoid pressure. *Anaesth Intensive Care* 1988;16:139–43

40. Mendelson CL. The aspiration of stomach contents into the lungs during obstetric anesthesia. *Am J Obstet Gynecol* 1946;52:191–204

41. Dewan DM, Writer WD, Wheeler AS, *et al.* Sodium citrate premedication in elective caesarean section patients. *Can Anaesth Soc J* 1982;29:355–8

42. Popat MT, Dyar OJ, Blogg CE. Comparison of the effects of oral nizatidine and ranitidine on gastric volume and pH in patients undergoing gynecological laparoscopy. *Anaesthesia* 1991;46:816–19

43. Suojaranta-Ylinen R, Hendolin H, Alhava E, Kontra K. The effect of prophylactic use of famotidine, ranitidine, and sodium citrate in upper abdominal surgery. *Agents Actions* 1990;30:297–9

44. Wren CA. An account of the rise and attempts of a way to convey liquors immediately into the mass of blood. *Philos Trans R Soc Lond* 1665;1:128–30

45. Thomas H Jr, Schwartz E, Petrilli R. Droperidol versus haloperidol for chemical restraint of agitated and combative patients. *Ann Emerg Med* 1992;21:407–13

46. Oré PC. Des injections intra-veineuses de chloral. *Paris Bull Soc Chir* 1872;1:400–12

47. Greenberg SB, Faerber EN, Aspinall CL. High dose chloral hydrate sedation for children undergoing CT. *J Comput Assist Tomogr* 1991;15:467–9

48. Rumm PD, Takao RT, Fox DJ, Atkinson SW. Efficacy of sedation of children with chloral hydrate. *South Med J* 1990;83:1040–3

49. Mirakhur RK, Dundee JW. Cardiovascular changes during induction of anaesthesia. Influence of three anticholinergic premedicants. *Ann R Coll Surg Engl* 1979;61:463–9

50. Braunn GG, Schywalsky M, Naujoks B, Brunner M, Danner U, Hauschild S. Atropine versus glycopyrrolate in eye surgery. A comparison of rhythm disorders and heart frequency using Holter-ECG [German]. *Anaesthesiol Reanim* 1992;17:57–65

51. Helfman SM, Gold MI, DeLisser EA, Herrington CA. Which drug prevents tachycardia and hypertension associated with tracheal intubation: lidocaine, fentanyl, or esmolol? *Anesth Analg* 1991;72:482–6

52. Kovac AL, Bennets PS, Ohara S, LaGreca BA, Khan JA, Calkins JW. Effect of esmolol on hemodynamics and intraocular pressure response to succinylcholine and intubation following low-dose alfentanil premedication. *J Clin Anesth* 1992;4:315–20

53. Liu PL, Gatt S, Gugino LD, Mallampati SR, Covino BG. Esmolol for control of increases in heart rate and blood pressure during tracheal intubation after thiopentone and succinylcholine. *Can Anaesth Soc J* 1986;33:556–62

54. Gaubatz CL, Wehner RJ. Evaluation of esmolol and fentanyl in controlling increases in heart rate and blood pressure during endotracheal intubation. *Am Assoc Nurse Anesth J* 1991;59:91–6

55. Inada E, Cullen DJ, Nemeskal AR, Teplick R. Effect of labetalol or lidocaine on the hemodynamic response to intubation: a controlled randomized double-blind study. *J Clin Anesth* 1989;1:207–13

56. Dahlgren G, Settergren G, Ohqvist G, Brodin LA. A comparative study of five different techniques to reduce left ventricular dysfunction during endotracheal intubation. *Acta Anaesthesiol Scand* 1991;35:609–15

57. Huguenard P, Dufeu N. Birth of neuroplegia and artificial hibernation in France. In Rupreht J, van Lieburg MJ, Lee JA, Erdmann W, eds. *Anaesthesia Essays on Its History*. Berlin, Heidelberg: Springer-Verlag, 1985:108–11

58. Randall LO, Heise GA, Schaller W, *et al*. Pharmacological and clinical studies on Valium™. A new psychotherapeutic agent of the benzodiazepine class. *Curr Ther Res* 1961;3:405–25

59. Huguenard P, Deligne P. Notes on the Taractan-Palfium-Gamma OH association with artificial ventilation in infantile neurosurgery. *Ann Anesthesiol Fr* 1965;6:315–18

60. Douit M. Diazepam in anesthesiology. Medical dissertation, University of Paris, 1965

61. Samuelson PN, Reves JG, Kouchoukos NT, Smith LR, Dole KM. Hemodynamic responses to anesthetic induction with midazolam or diazepam in patients with ischemic heart disease. *Anesth Analg* 1981;60:802–9

62. Tateishi A, Maekawa T, Takeshita H, Wakuta K. Diazepam and intracranial pressure. *Anesthesiology* 1981;54:335–7

63. Henry DW, Burwinkle JW, Klutman NE. Determination of sedative and amnestic doses of lorazepam in children. *Clin Pharm* 1991;10:625–9

64. Sievers TD, Yee JD, Foley ME, Blanding PJ, Berde CB. Midazolam for conscious sedation during pediatric oncology procedures: safety and recovery parameters. *Pediatrics* 1991;88:1172–9

65. Wright SW, Chudnofsky CR, Dronen SC, Wright MB, Borron SW. Midazolam use in the emergency department. *Am J Emerg Med* 1990;8:97–100

66. Bailey PL, Pace NL, Ashburn MA, Moll JWB, East KA, Stanley TH. Frequent hypoxemia and apnea after sedation with midazolam and fentanyl. *Anesthesiology* 1990;73:826–30

67. Nishiyama T, Hirasaki A, Odaka Y, Seto K, Goto I. Midazolam for rapid sequence induction [Japanese]. *Masui – Jpn J Anesthesiol* 1990;39:230–6

68. Bartholow R. *Manual of Hypodermic Medication*, 2nd edn. Philadelphia: JB Lippincott, 1873:1–170

69. Brederfeld E. Die intravenose narkose mit arzneigemischen. *F Exp Path Ther* 1916;18:80–90

70. Chudnofsky CR, Wright SW, Dronen SC, Borron SW, Wright MB. The safety of fentanyl use in the emergency department. *Ann Emerg Med* 1989;18:635–9

71. From RP, Warner DS, Todd MM, Sokoll MD. Anesthesia for craniotomy: a double-blind comparison of alfentanil, fentanyl and sufentanil. *Anesthesiology* 1990;73:896–904

72. Saltanov AI, Kadyrova EG, Lunevskii VI, Remez VF, Goloskov NP. An evaluation of the effect of certain factors on the hemodynamics during anesthesia induction in stomach cancer patients [Russian]. *Anesteziol Reanimatol* 1990;1:3–6

73. Chraemmer-Jorgensen B, Hertel S, Strom J, Hoilund-Carlsen PF, Bjerre-Jepsen K. Catecholamine response to laryngoscopy and intubation. The influence of three different drug combinations commonly used for induction of anaesthesia. *Anaesthesia* 1992;47:750–6

74. Zerfas LG, McCallum JTL, Shorle HA, *et al*. Induction of anesthesia in man by the intravenous injection of sodium-ISO-amyl-ethyl barbiturate. *Proc Soc Exp Biol Med* 1929;26:399–403

75. Lundy JS. The barbiturates as anesthetics, hypnotics and antispasmodics: their use in more than 1000 surgical and nonsurgical

clinical cases and in operations on animals. *Anesth Analg* 1929;8:360–5

76. Lundy JS. Intravenous anesthesia: preliminary report of the use of two new thiobarbiturates. *Proc Staff Meet Mayo Clin* 1935;10:536–43

77. Giffin JP, Cottrell JE, Shwiry B, Hartung J, Epstein J, Lim K. Intracranial pressure, mean arterial pressure and heart rate following midazolam or thiopental in humans with brain tumors. *Anesthesiology* 1984;60:491–4

78. Alvarez Gomez JA, Estelles Montesinos ME, Palacios Sanchez MA. Comparison of the effects of midazolam and thiopental on the neuromuscular response of vecuronium, atracurium, and pancuronium [Spanish]. *Rev Esp Anestesiol Reanim* 1991;38:293–6

79. Zink BJ, Darfler K, Salluzzo RF, Reilly KM. The efficacy and safety of methohexital in the emergency department. *Ann Emerg Med* 1991; 20:1293–8

80. Kruger AD, Benad G. The treatment of status asthmaticus using ketamine – experimental results and clinical experience [German]. *Anaesthesiol Reanim* 1992;17:109–30

81. White PF, Way WL, Trevor AJ. Ketamine – its pharmacology and therapeutic uses. *Anesthesiology* 1982;56:119–36

82. Cartwright PD, Pingel SM. Midazolam and diazepam in ketamine anaesthesia. *Anaesthesia* 1984;39:439–42

83. Pfenninger E, Dick W, Ahnefeld FW. The influence of ketamine on both normal and raised intracranial pressure of artificially ventilated animals. *Eur J Anesth* 1985;2: 297–307

84. Paulin M, Jullian-Papouin H, Roquebert PO, Manelli JC. Hemodynamic effects of propofol used alone for the induction of anesthesia [French]. *Ann Fr Anesth Reanim* 1987;6:237–9

85. Coley S, Mobley KA, Bone ME, Fell D. Hemodynamic changes after induction of anaesthesia and tracheal intubation following propofol or thiopentone in patients of ASA grade I and III. *Br J Anaesth* 1989;63: 423–8

86. Giese JL, Stanley TH. Etomidate: a new intravenous anesthetic induction agent. *Pharmacotherapy* 1983;3:251–8

87. Giese JL, Stockham RJ, Stanley TH, Pace NL, Nelissen RH. Etomidate versus thiopental for induction of anesthesia. *Anesth Analg* 1985;64: 871–6

88. Thomas B, Meirlaen L, Rolly G, Weyne L. Clinical use of etomidate. *Acta Anaesthesiol Belg* 1976;27:167–74

89. Snow J. On the inhalation of the vapour of ether. *Lond Med Gaz* 1847;39:498–502

90. Worthington ED. Cases of chloroform. *Br Am J Med Phys Sci* 1848;3:326–7

91. Hewitt F. The administration of nitrous oxide and ether in combination or succession. *Br Med J* 1887;2:452–4

92. Stiles JA, Neff WB, Povenstine EA, Waters RM. Cyclopropane as an anesthetic agent. *Curr Res Anesth Analg* 1934;13:56–60

93. Arky R, ed. *Physicians' Desk Reference*, 48th edn. Notvale, NJ: Medical Economics Data Production Company, 1994

94. Griffith HR, Johnson GE. The use of curine in general anesthesia. *Anesthesiology* 1942;3: 418–20

95. Scurr CF. Use of suxamethonium iodide in anesthesia for peroneal endoscopy. *Br Med J* 1950;2:1311

96. Forbes AR, Cohen NH, Eger EI. Pancuronium reduces halothane requirement in man. *Anesth Analg* 1979;54:497–9

97. DeGarmo BH, Dronen S. Pharmacology and clinical use of neuromuscular blocking agents. *Ann Emerg Med* 1983;12:48–55

98. Bruton-Maree N. Neuromuscular blocking drugs. *J Neurosci Nurs* 1989;21:198–200

99. Talucci RC, Shaik KA, Schwab CW. Rapid sequence induction with oral endotracheal intubation in the multiply injured patient. *Am Surg* 1988;54:185–7

100. Cicala R, Westbrook L. An alternative method of paralysis for rapid-sequence induction. *Anesthesiology* 1988;69:983–6

101. Gorback MS, Graubert DA. Gastroesophageal reflux during anesthetic induction with thiopental and succinylcholine. *J Clin Anesth* 1990;2:163–7

102. Salem MR, Wong AY, Lin YH. The effect of suxamethonium on the intragastric pressure in infants and children. *Br J Anaesth* 1972;44: 16–19

103. Sosis M, Broad T, Larijani GE, Marr AT. Comparison of atracurium and *d*-tubo-curarine for prevention of succinylcholine myalgia. *Anesth Analg* 1987;66:657–9

104. Joshi C, Bruce DL. Thiopental and succinylcholine: action on intraocular pressure. *Anesth Analg* 1975;54:471–5

105. Libonati MM, Leahy JJ, Ellison N. The use of succinylcholine in open eye surgery. *Anesthesiology* 1983;62:637–40

106. Keneally JP, Bush GH. Changes in serum potassium after suxamethonium in children. *Anaesth Intensive Care* 1974;2:147–50

107. Van Der Spek AFL, Fang WB, Ashton-Miller JA, Stohler CS, Carlson DS, Schork MA. The effects of succinylcholine on mouth opening. *Anesthesiology* 1987;67:459–65

108. Minton MD, Grosslight K, Stirt JA, Bedford RF. Increases in intracranial pressure from succinylcholine: prevention by prior non-depolarizing blockade. *Anesthesiology* 1986;65: 165–9

109. Kovarik WD, Mayber TS, Lam AM, Mathisen TL, Winn HR. Succinylcholine does not change intracranial pressure, cerebral blood flow velocity or the electroencephalogram in patients with neurologic injury. *Anesth Analg* 1994;78:469–73

110. Kunjappan VE, Brown EM, Alexander GD. Rapid sequence induction using vecuronium. *Anesth Analg* 1986;65:503–6

111. Huemer G, Schwarz S, Gilly H, Weindlmayr-Goettel M, Plainer B, Lackner F. Pharmacodynamics, pharmacokinetics, and intubation conditions after priming with three different doses of vecuronium. *Anesth Analg* 1995;80:538–42

112. Davison KL, Holland MS. A comparison study of vecuronium bromide and atracurium besylate for rapid sequence induction. *J Am Assoc Nurse Anesth* 1989;57:37–40

113. Silverman DG, Swift CA, Dubow HD, O'Connor TZ, Brull SJ. Variability of onset times within and among relaxant regimens. *J Clin Anesth* 1992;4:28–33

114. Mortier E, Versichelen L, Herregods L, Rolly G. Priming with vecuronium and atracurium – a comparison. *Acta Anaesthesiol Belg* 1987; 38:83–7

115. Yamada T, Takino Y. A single bolus dose of vecuronium for rapid endotracheal intubation [Japanese]. *Masui – Jpn J Anesthesiol* 1992; 41:15–18

116. Mirakhur RK. Newer neuromuscular blocking drugs. An overview of their clinical pharmacology and therapeutic use. *Drugs* 1992;44:182–99

117. Schaer H, Baasch K, Nassehi R. Comparative clinical studies of vecuronium, atracurium and pancuronium [German]. *Anaesthetist* 1984;33:259–65

118. Payne JP, Hughes R. Evaluation of atracurium in anaesthetized man. *Br J Anaesth* 1981;53:45–54

119. Miller RD, Rupp SM, Fisher DM, Cronnelly R, Fahey MR, Sohn YJ. Clinical pharmacology of vecuronium and atracurium. *Anesthesiology* 1984;61:444–53

120. Goudsouzian NG, Liu LM, Cote CJ. Comparison of equipotent doses of nondepolarizing muscle relaxants in children. *Anesth Analg* 1981;60:862–6

121. Johnstone M, Mahmoud AA, Mrozinski RA. Cardiovascular effects of tubocurarine in man. *Anaesthesia* 1978;33:587–93

122. Williams A, Gyasi H, Melloni C, Bevan DR. Clinical experience with ORG NC45 (Norcuron) as the sole muscle relaxant. *Can Anaesth Soc J* 1982;29:567–72

123. Forstmann V, Schuh FT. Onset of the effect and intubation conditions following atracurium, vecuronium and suxamethonium [German]. *Anaesthetist* 1988;37:311–15

124. Ueda N, Muteki T, Tsuda H, Masuda Y, Ohishi K, Tobata H. Determining the optimal time for endotracheal intubation during onset of neuromuscular blockade. *Eur J Anesthesiol* 1993;10:3–8

125. Deepika K, Bikhazi GB, Mikati HM, Namba M, Foldes FF. Facilitation of rapid-sequence intubation with large-dose vecuronium with or without priming. *J Clin Anesth* 1992;4: 106–10

126. Khuenl-Brady KS, Scharz S, Richardson FJ, Mitterschiffthaler G. Maintenance of surgical muscle relaxation by repeat doses of vecuronium and atracurium at three different dose levels. *Eur J Anesth* 1991;8: 1–6

127. Koller ME, Husby P. High-dose vecuronium may be an alternative to suxamethonium for rapid-sequence intubation. *Acta Anaesthesiol Scand* 1993;37:465–8

128. Gergis SD, Sokoll MD, Mehta M, Kemmotsu O, Rudd GD. Intubation conditions after atracurium and suxamethonium. *Br J Anaesth* 1983;55:83S–86S

129. Luyk NH, Weaver JM, Quinn C, Wilson S, Beck FM. Comparative trial of succinyl-choline vs low dose atracurium–lidocaine combination for intubation in short out-patient procedures. *Anesth Prog* 1990;37: 238–43

130. Famewo CE. Conditions for endotracheal intubation after atracurium and suxamethonium. *Mid East J Anesthesiol* 1986;8:371–7

131. Hunter JM, Jones RS, Utting JE. Use of atracurium in patients with no renal function. *Br J Anaesth* 1982;54:1251–8

132. Cardone C, Szenohradszky J, Yost S, Bickler PE. Activation of brain acetylcholine receptors by neuromuscular blocking drugs. A possible mechanism of neurotoxicity. *Anesthesiology* 1994;80:1155–61

133. Katz Y, Weizman A, Pick CG, *et al.* Interactions between laudanosine, GABA, and opioid subtype receptors: implication for laudanosine seizure activity. *Brain Res* 1994; 646:235–41

134. Roizen MF, Feeley TW. Pancuronium bromide. *Ann Intern Med* 1978;88:64–8

135. Mehta MP, Choi WW, Gergis SD, Sokoll MD, Adolphson AJ. Facilitation of rapid endotracheal intubations with divided doses of nondepolarizing neuromuscular blocking drugs. *Anesthesiology* 1985;62:392–5

136. Montgomery CJ, Steward DJ. A comparative evaluation of intubating doses of atracurium, *d*-tubocurarine, pancuronium and vecuronium in children. *Can J Anaesth* 1988;35:36–40

137. Twohig MM, Ward S, Corall IM. Conditions for tracheal intubation using atracurium compared with pancuronium. *Br J Anaesth* 1983;55:87S–89S

138. Frampton JE, McTavish D. Mivacurium. A review of its pharmacology and therapeutic potential in general anaesthesia. *Drugs* 1993;45:1066–89

139. Savarese JJ, Ali HH, Basta SJ, *et al.* The clinical neuromuscular pharmacology of mivacurium chloride (BW B1090U). A short-acting nondepolarizing ester neuromuscular blocking drug. *Anesthesiology* 1988;68:723–32

140. Goldberg ME, Larijani GE, Azad SS, *et al.* Comparison of tracheal intubating conditions and neuromuscular blocking profiles after intubating doses of mivacurium chloride or succinylcholine in surgical outpatients. *Anesth Analg* 1989;69:93–9

141. Mangat PS, Evans DE, Harmer M, Lunn JN. A comparison between mivacurium and suxamethonium in children. *Anaesthesia* 1993; 48:866–90

142. Wierda JM, Hommes FD, Nap HJ, van den Broek L. Time course of action and intubating conditions following vecuronium, rocuronium and mivacurium. *Anaesthesia* 1995;50:393–6

143. Magorian T, Wood P, Caldwell J, *et al.* The pharmacokinetics and neuromuscular effects of rocuronium bromide in patients with liver disease. *Anesth Analg* 1995;80:754–9

144. Khuenl-Brady KS, Pomaroli A, Puhringer F, Mitterschiffthaler G, Koller J. The use of rocuronium (ORG 9426) in patients with chronic renal failure. *Anaesthesia* 1993;48: 873–5

145. Huizinga AC, Vandenbrom RH, Wierda JM, Hommes FD, Hennis PJ. Intubating conditions and onset of neuromuscular block of rocuronium (Org 9426); a comparison with suxamethonium. *Acta Anaesthesiol Scan*d 1992; 36:463–8

146. De Mey JC, Debrock M, Rolly G. Evaluation of the onset and intubation conditions of rocuronium bromide. *Eur J Anesth* 1994;9:37–40

147. Dubois MY, Lea DE, Kataria B, Gadde PL, Tran DQ, Shearrow T. Pharmacodynamics of rocuronium with and without prior administration of succinylcholine. *J Clin Anesth* 1995; 7:44–8

148. Puhringer FK, Khuenl-Brady KS, Koller J, Mitterschiffthaler G. Evaluation of the endotracheal intubating conditions of rocuronium (ORG 9426) and succinylcholine in outpatient surgery. *Anesth Analg* 1992; 75:37–40

149. Magorian T, Flannery KB, Miller RD. Comparison of rocuronium, succinylcholine and vecuronium for rapid sequence induction of anesthesia in adult patients. *Anesthesiology* 1993;79:913–18

150. Crul JF, Vanbelleghem V, Buyse L, Heylen R, van Egmond J. Rocuronium with alfentanil and propofol allows intubation within 45 seconds. *Eur J Anesth* 1995;11:111–12

151. Tryba M, Zorn A, Thole H, Zenz M. Rapid-sequence orotracheal intubation with rocuronium: a randomized double-blind comparison with suxamethonium – preliminary communication. *Eur J Anesth* 1994;9:44–8

152. Welch RM, Brown A, Ravitch J, Dahl R. The *in vitro* degradation of cisatracurium, the R, *cis*-R′-isomer of atracurium, in human and rat plasma. *Clin Pharmacol Ther* 1995;58:132–42

153. Konstadt SN, Reich DL, Stanley TE 3rd, *et al.* A two-center comparison of the cardiovascular effects of cisatracurium (Nimbex) and vecuronium in patients with coronary artery disease. *Anesth Analg* 1995;81: 1010–14

154. Prielipp RC, Coursin DB, Scuderi PE, *et al.* Comparison of the infusion requirements and recovery profiles of vecuronium and cisatracurium 51W89 in intensive care unit patients. *Anesth Analg* 1995;81:3–12

155. Moore CD, Klasco R, eds. *Micro Medex System*. Englewood, Co: Medex, 2000

156. Product information. Raplon™. 1999

157. Donati F, McCarroll SM, Antzake C, McCready D, Bevan DR. Dose–response curves for edrophonium, neostigmine and pyridostigmine after pancuronium and *d*-tubocurarine. *Anesthesiology* 1987;66:471–6

158. Hannington-Kiff JG. Timing of atropine and neostigmine in the reversal of muscle relaxants. *Br Med J* 1969;1:418–20

159. Larach DR, Hensley FA Jr, Martin DE, High KM, Rung GW, Skeehan TM. Hemodynamic effects of muscle relaxant drugs during anesthetic induction in patients with mitral or aortic valvular heart disease. *J Cardiothorac Vasc Anesth* 1991;5:126–31

160. Sethna DH, Staff NJ, Estafanous FG. Cardiovascular effects of non-depolarizing neuromuscular blockers in patients with coronary artery disease. *Can Anaesth Soc J* 1986;33:280–6

161. Redan JA, Livingston DH, Tortella BJ, Rush BF Jr. The value of intubating and paralyzing patients with suspected head injury in the emergency department. *J Trauma* 1991;31: 371–5

162. Ligier B, Buchman TG, Breslow MJ, Deutschman CS. The role of anesthetic induction agents and neuromuscular blockade in the endotracheal intubation of trauma victims. *Surg Gynecol Obstet* 1991; 173:477–81

163. Syverud SA, Borron SW, Storer DL. Prehospital use of neuromuscular blocking agents in a helicopter ambulance program. *Ann Emerg Med* 1988;17:236–42

164. Greenbaum R, Cooper R, Hulme A, Mackintosh IP. The effect of induction of anaesthesia on intracranial pressure. In Arias A, ed. *Recent Progress in Anesthesiology and Resuscitation*. Amsterdam: Exerpta Medica, 1975

165. Burney RG, Winn R. Increased cerebrospinal fluid pressure during laryngoscopy and intubation or induction of anesthesia. *Anesth Analg* 1975;54:687–90

166. Rosa G, Sanfilippo M, Vilardi V, Orfei P, Gasparetto A. Effects of vecuronium bromide on intracranial pressure and cerebral perfusion pressure. *Br J Anaesth* 1986;58:437–40

167. Rosa G, Orfei P, Sanfilippo M, Vilardi V, Gasparetto A. The effects of atracurium besylate (Tracrium) on intracranial pressure and cerebral perfusion pressure. *Anesth Analg* 1986;65:381–4

168. Meschino A, Devitt JH, Koch JP, Szalai JP, Schwartz ML. The safety of awake tracheal intubation in cervical spine injury. *Can J Anaesth* 1992;39:114–17

169. Suderman VS, Crosby ET, Lui A. Elective oral tracheal intubation in cervical spine-injured adults. *Can J Anesth* 1991;38:785–9

170. Rhee KJ, Green W, Holcroft JW, Mangili JAA. Oral intubation in the multiply injured patient: the risk of exacerbating spinal cord damage. *Ann Emerg Med* 1990;19:511–14

171. Hauswald M, Sklar DP, Tandberg D, Garcia JF. Cervical spine movement during airway management: cinefluoroscopic appraisal in human cadavers. *Am J Emerg Med* 1991;9:535–8

172. Majernick TG, Bieniek R, Houston JB, Hughes HG. Cervical spine movement during orotracheal intubation. *Ann Emerg Med* 1986;15:417–20

173. Aprahamian C, Thompson BM, Finger WA, Darin JC. Experimental cervical spine injury model: evaluation of airway management and splinting techniques. *Ann Emerg Med* 1984; 13:584–7

174. Bivins HG, Ford S, Bezmalinovic Z, Price HM, Williams JL. The effect of axial traction during orotracheal intubation of the trauma victim with an unstable cervical spine. *Ann Emerg Med* 1988;17:25–9

175. Scannell G, Waxman K, Tominaga G, Barker S, Anna C. Orotracheal intubation in trauma patients with cervical fractures. *Arch Surg* 1993;128:903–6

176. Eggen JT, Jorgen RC. Airway management, penetrating neck trauma. *J Emerg Med* 1993; 11:381–5

177. Schaner PJ, Brown RL, Kirksey TD, Gunther RC, Ritchey CR, Gronert GA. Succinylcholine-induced hyperkalemia in burned patients – 1. *Anesth Analg* 1969;48:764–70

178. Gronert GA, Theye RA. Pathophysiology of hyperkalemia induced by succinylcholine. *Anesthesiology* 1975;43:89–97

179. van Beem H, Manger FW, van Boxtel C, van Bentem N. Etomidate anaesthesia in patients with cirrhosis of the liver: pharmacokinetic data. *Anaesthesia* 1983;38:61–2

Difficult tracheal intubation: prediction, assessment and intervention

2

INTRODUCTION

Laryngoscopy and intubation have been described by Flagg as 'the pivot upon which turns the movement to prevent asphyxial death'[1]. This quote effectively captures the essence of this crucial procedure, which balances between safe airway control and failed intubation.

The irony is that most situations encountered are routine and accomplished easily using standardized approaches. The minority of cases – the so-called difficult intubation scenarios – consume most of the thought and effort devoted to study of intubation accompanied by failed ventilation. A literature review has compiled the current standards of care regarding a difficult airway: predisposed populations, prediction tools, methods of assessment, laryngoscope review, intubation techniques and modified surgical approaches to airway control.

History

The modern resurgence of endotracheal intubation began with the reintroduction of this device for administration of anesthesia by MacEwen in 1880[2]. Jackson developed an early laryngoscope in 1907; this was a hollow device similar to a rigid bronchoscope for operative intubation[3]. Clinical use of laryngoscopy and endotracheal intubation for airway control was described in 1913[4].

Today's laryngoscope has its roots in a double-bladed intubation device designed by d'Etoille in 1827 for laryngeal tube insertion and described in the *Journal de Recherches sur l'Asphyxie*[5]. Modern laryngoscope development began in the early 1940s. The most popular designs were the Miller device, a straight blade with a curved tip, and the MacIntosh blade, which is curved throughout its length[6,7].

Education

Teaching intubation skills may be especially problematic, considering the emergency nature of the intervention, the incidence of difficult airway and the significant sequelae associated with esophageal intubation.

Emergency intubation in 779 patients studied by Stewart and colleagues[8] was associated with a 90% success rate in the prehospital setting, with 58% correct placement on the first attempt, 26% on the second attempt and only 5% on the third attempt. The incidence of undiagnosed esophageal intubation in routine practice is minimal (0.38%) based on this series[8]. Gabram and co-workers suggested that additional caution is warranted when intubating trauma patients. They had an initial success rate of 93%, although pharmacological induction strategies resulted in successful intubation in all 106 cases studied[9].

Teaching difficult intubation skills requires recognition and anticipation of known problematic situations, such as with emergency or trauma patients, or patients with anatomic abnormalities. The learning curve may be steep, as described in an antiquated training model attributed to Chevalier Jackson[10], describing the beginning point with the first intubation, the practitioner able to make positional changes by 100 procedures, to make technique changes by 1000 and to teach improvisational technique modification to others only when 10 000 successful intubations had been completed.

Jackson also contributed the statement that 'endoscopic ability cannot be bought with the instruments. As with all mechanical procedures, facility can be obtained only by education, the eye, and the fingers in repeated exercise of a particular series of maneuvers. As with learning to play a musical instrument, a fundamental knowledge of technique, positions and landmarks is necessary, after which only continued manual practice makes for proficiency'[11].

Successful training strategies for instruction in intubation technique use a multimodal approach. In Stewart's study of 146 emergency medical service personnel, initial intubation success was enhanced by the use of didactic sessions and manikin training programs (77%), improved to 84% by the addition of animal models, improved to 88% with human operating room cases, and successful in 95% of those cases performed by operators achieving preceptor status[12]. Training strategies for anesthesia residents using a simulated difficult intubation compared to a standard intubation model found no difference in cardiopulmonary parameters (heart rate, blood pressure or oxygen saturation), but a 25% esophageal intubation rate in the difficult intubation training group demonstrated in the evaluation of 40 patient simulations by Goldberg and associates[13].

Clinical data suggested that multiple intubation attempts were required for 18% of patients encountered in a sample of 1195 cases, mostly due to operator inexperience[10]. Although inappropriate blade choice is often invoked as a cause of failed intubation, a laryngoscope blade change is usually successful in only 4% of patients[10]. The presence of an organized systematic approach to intubation is more important than the individual technique utilized.

The difficult airway, designated by inability to visualize the larynx, resulting in unsuccessful intubation, is an infrequent (1–4%) but critical occurrence[14–16]. Preoperative airway evaluation should include a careful exploration of history of prior difficulty with intubation or excessive snoring, and proper use of anatomic measurements, physical examination and preoperative testing, such as dynamic fluoroscopy, if indicated[14]. This systematic approach may help avoid errors, such as positional abnormalities, and provide for assessment of adequate oral excursion, proper blade insertion, vocal cord exposure and endotracheal tube (ETT) introduction under direct visualization[17]. Training should include adequate instruction, simulation sessions, practice models and controlled clinical experience with patients.

ANESTHETIC MISADVENTURE

The incidence of difficult intubation is small (0.13%) but problematic, because it is not anticipated in 10–53% of patients in which it is encountered[18,19]. Difficult intubation is often predicted by the presence of obesity, short neck, oropharyngeal tumor, temporomandibular joint ankylosis, cervical ankylosis, maxillofacial deformity, or cervical fracture[18]. Unexpected difficulties arise in those with limited oral excursion, elongated incisors, a rigid epiglottis, or excessive muscle relaxation[18].

Anesthetic misadventure was described in the American Society of Anesthesiology Closed Claims Project in 2046 cases collected from events occurring between 1974 and 1987[20]. These events were of respiratory origin in one-third (37%) of the cases, and were associated with difficult intubation, esophageal intubation, or inadequate ventilation, resulting in severe brain injury or death in 47% of cases[20].

In a similar analysis, based on the Canadian Anesthesia Society survey of 2000 anesthetists over 7 years, 602 accidents were reported with esophageal intubations in one-third of patients and accidents with identifiable error in technique in half of the cases resulting in death or cerebral damage[21].

An analysis by Craig and Wilson of 8000 cases found an 0.97% incidence of anesthesia complications. These complications were due to human error in two-thirds of cases and equipment failure in 12% of patients[22]. A 4% incidence of difficult intubation was reported in an Australian Incident Monitoring Study of 2000 problematic cases, where one-third of these difficult intubations were emergency cases, one-third involved an unassisted trainee and over 20% occurred outside normal working hours[15].

Beinlich described an anesthetic case mortality rate of 1 : 10 000 due to difficult intubation, aspiration, hypoventilation, volume overload, or cardiac dysfunction specifically occurring in 10% of all patients[23]. Factors correlated with complications during anesthesia include patient age, co-morbid disease, anesthesia technique and level of experience of operator[23].

Specific patient populations, such as those requiring obstetric care, deserve special note. Lyons' survey of 2500 obstetric anesthesia cases evaluated over a 6-year period demonstrated a 1 in 300 failed intubation rate with no retrospective maxillofacial abnormalities noted[24]. An evaluation by Jay and associates included drug overdose patients, with 77% of patients requiring intubation; 10% of these intubations were rated as difficult[25]. Subsequent mortality in 195 of these patients was associated with aspiration (94%), pulmonary infiltrate (44%), or increased ventilatory requirement (43%)[25].

CONDITIONS

A wide variety of anatomic, physiological and pathological conditions are associated with intubation difficulty (Table 1)[26–48]. Obstetric patients can be predisposed to difficulty, because of tissue swelling, laryngeal edema due to the Valsalva maneuver occurring during labor, pre-eclampsia, prominent breast and redundant oropharyngeal soft tissue[26].

Cervical spine injury is one of the most difficult intubation scenarios. Patients with unstable cervical injury often have neurological deficit (33%) and undergo oral intubation (71%) facilitated by pharmacological induction (55%)[27]. Cervical immobilization was documented by Suderman and colleagues in only half of a series of 150 patients[27]. These patients had a new neurological deficit in 1.3% of cases, with no correlation noted on whether nasal or oral intubation was used[27]. The placement of a rigid cervical collar,

Table 1 Conditions associated with difficult intubation[26–48]

Pregnancy
Cervical spine injury
Burns
Pseudoxanthoma elasticum
Pemphigoid
Mucopolysaccharidosis
Stylohyoid ligament calcification
Carotid endarterectomy
Neck abscess
Obesity
Temporomandibular joint dysfunction
Laryngeal web
Tumor
Mandibular hypoplasia
Treacher–Collins syndrome
Pierre–Robin syndrome
Cherubism
Stiff man syndrome
Acromegaly
Cervical spondylosis
Arthritis
Diffuse idiopathic skeletal hyperostosis

although protective, itself makes intubation difficult, with mouth opening reduced by as much as 60% in some cases[28].

The burned patient is plagued acutely by airway swelling and chronically by limited mobility due to scarring. Flexible bronchoscopically guided nasal intubation was successful in 15 of 17 burn patients studied by Larson and Parks[29]. Patients with pseudoxanthoma elasticum often have a rigid epiglottis resulting in difficulty with vocal cord visualization, which can be facilitated by bronchoscopic guidance[30]. Those with pemphigoid also have connective tissue involvement causing a stenotic laryngeal orifice, which may be circumvented by flexible stylet placement[31] (Figure 1).

Mucopolysaccharidosis, a type of connective tissue-manufacturing defect that presents in pediatric patients, was associated with a difficult airway incidence in one-quarter of cases with an intubation failure rate of three in 34 patients[32]. Difficult airway in 54% and failed intubation incidence of 23% were reported with Hurler's syndrome, a particularly problematic disorder[32].

Calcification of the stylohyoid ligament connecting the temporal to the hyoid bones results in laryngeal immobility restricting lateral movement to 1.5 cm or less, which often hinders successful intubation[33]. This condition may be diagnosed by a skin crease over the hyoid bone, indicative of a rigid fixed epiglottis and often requiring bronchoscopic intubation[34].

The association of head and neck surgery and difficult airway is well established. Carotid endarterectomy patients are frequently afflicted with soft tissue swelling and hematoma[35]. The 'air-leak test', wherein successful extubation is predicted by the presence of an audible air leak with the endotracheal tube deflated, is suggested in these cases (Figure 2).

Potgieter and Hammond[36] described the 'cuff-leak test', wherein the cuff pressure is released and the ETT digitally included. If air movement is audible, the patient may be safely extubated in the setting of laryngeal edema, on the basis of a clinical trial of ten patients. Fisher and Raper evaluated an initial group of 62 patients with upper airway obstruction[37]. All 55 of those with a cuff leak were successfully extubated, whereas all of those who failed serial tests required reintubation ($n = 2$) or underwent tracheostomy ($n = 5$)[37]. The follow-up study evaluated ten cases of those who failed the cuff-leak test, and found that the majority (seven cases) were successfully extubated, while three required subsequent tracheostomy[37]. Thus, the cuff-leak test is sensitive but not specific in predicting extubation success, in that those who leak may be successfully extubated,

whereas those who do not leak may not necessarily fail and require reintubation.

The presence of a deep neck abscess is associated with significant mortality, which was found to decrease from 50 to 5% with improvements in therapy over time[38]. Classification proceeds by location – diffuse, suprahyoid, or infrahyoid – and intubation may be attempted with clear visualization of the oropharynx, whereas tracheostomy is more prudent with severe involvement or suspicion of obstruction (Figure 3).

The presence of obesity with resulting airway soft tissue redundancy and limitations on patient positioning by stature can be problematic[39]. Additional correlatives include poor cardiac reserve due to accompanying hypertension, diabetes mellitus and lack of exercise (Figure 4).

Temporomandibular joint dysfunction, such as 'pseudo ankylosis', occasionally requires surgery and may be complicated by hematoma, scarring and contracture, resulting in unilateral immobility interfering with subsequent intubation attempts[40] (Figure 5). The laryngeal web is an asymptomatic vocal cord

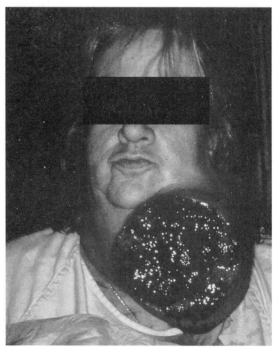

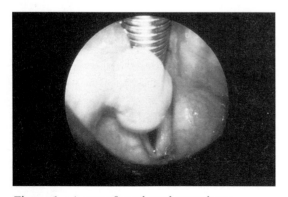

Figure 1   A case of vocal cord granuloma

Figure 2   Head and neck malignancy

scar, which is often the result of a prior injury[41]. This condition is difficult to diagnose and flow-volume loop testing is often normal[41]. The presence of a laryngeal web is addressed with laser therapy or by bronchoscopically guided nasal intubation. The presence of benign or malignant oropharyngeal lesions is a predisposing factor to physical obstruction or bleeding. Mortality with structural airway obstruction refractory to an intubation attempt has been described[42].

Congenital mandibular hypoplasia conditions such as Treacher–Collins or Pierre–Robin syndrome are common difficult intubation scenarios (Figure 6). These readily identifiable external abnormalities are characterized by hemifacial microsomia, macroglossia, glossoptosis, trismus and prominent maxillary incisors, and they can be addressed with otolaryngology assistance using the Jackson anterior commissure laryngoscope if conventional intubation attempts fail[43] (Figures 7 and 8). Cherubism characterized by maxillary and mandibular enlargement with an 'eyes to heaven' appearance often benefits from nasotracheal or fiberoptic intubation strategies[44] (Figure 9).

The stiff joint syndrome, characterized by diabetes mellitus, non-familial short stature, joint contractures and atlanto-occipital immobility, also requires fiberoptic intubation[45]. Patients with acromegaly demonstrate chondrocalcinosis, laryngeal calcification, and a large immobile obstructing epiglottis associated with poor vocal cord visualization[46].

Arthritis, especially rheumatoid conditions, is associated with cervical spondylosis, osteophyte enlargement, disk rigidity and esophageal distortion, making both positioning and laryngeal visualization difficult[47]. Diffuse idiopathic skeletal hyperostosis is often associated with anterior cervical osteophytes and posterior longitudinal ligament calcification, resulting in superior tracheal displacement[48] (Figures 10 and 11).

ASSESSMENT

Morphological features associated with difficult intubation include a short neck, full dentition,

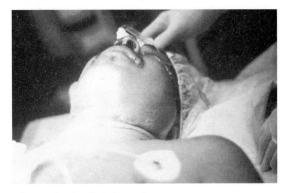

Figure 3 Ludwig's angina

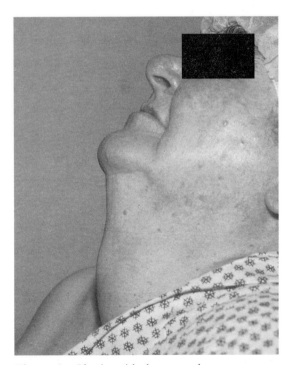

Figure 4 Obesity with thyromegaly

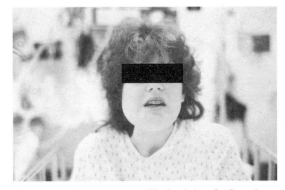

Figure 5 Temporomandibular joint dysfunction

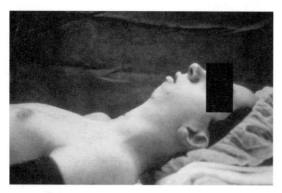

Figure 6   Retrognathia

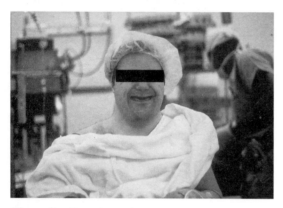

Figure 7   Down's syndrome

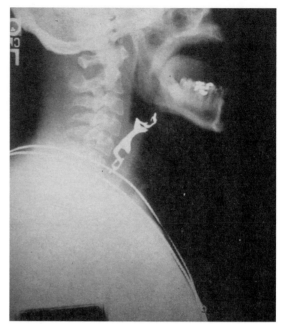

Figure 8   Displaced dental plate

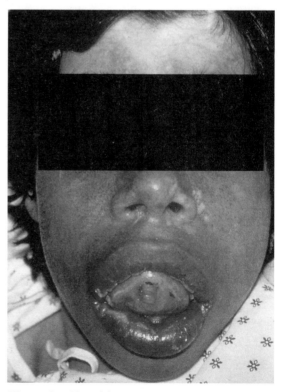

Figure 9   Cherubism

receding mandible, protruding maxilla, poor mandibular mobility, high palate and an increased alveolar–mental distance[49]. In a population with intubations categorized as not difficult, anticipated difficult, and not anticipated difficult, mandible length and depth, as well as the thyromental distance measured between the symphysis mentis and thyroid cartilage were found to be predictive of subsequent intubation difficulty[50] (Figure 12).

Although an extremely anterior larynx is the most commonly invoked reason for intubation failure, the most important aspect of endotracheal intubation may rather be adequate assessment, in both elective and emergency situations[51]. Assessment begins with an adequate history, emphasizing prior difficulty with intubation, airway-obstructive symptoms or prior need for a surgical airway. Physical examination of oropharyngeal structures should always be performed under elective conditions and if possible under emergency conditions (Figure 13).

Mallampati hypothesized that the ease of exposure of oral structures including the tongue, palatoglossal and palatopharyngeal pillars, and the uvula correlates with the ease of intubation[52]. The Mallampati classification system[53], based on evaluation of 210 patients, specifies class I (74%) as all structures visible, class II (19%) as facial pillars and soft palate visible, and class III (7%) as only soft palate visible, associated with a high false-positive rate and a low positive predictive value (Figure 14).

Cormack and Lehane developed a direct laryngoscopy grading system for obstetric patients[54]. In grade I, the glottis is visualized in 99% of intubations; in grade II, the posterior glottis is visualized in 1%; in grade III (1 in 2000), the epiglottis but not the vocal cords is identified; and in grade IV (1 in 10 000 cases), even the epiglottis is not visualized (Figure 15).

The Mallampati and Cormack scales have been validated as accurate predictors of intubation success ($p < 0.001$) in the operating room setting (Table 2)[52-54]. The Mallampati class I patients were associated with Cormack grade I (81%) or grade II (19%) laryngoscopy,

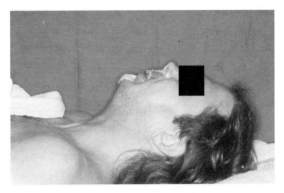

Figure 12 Occult difficult airway

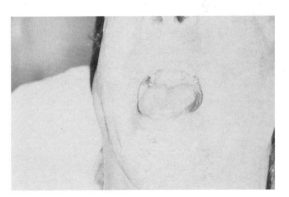

Figure 13 Decreased oral excursion

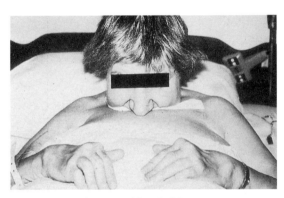

Figure 10 Rheumatoid arthritis

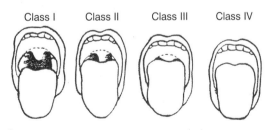

Class I   Class II   Class III   Class IV

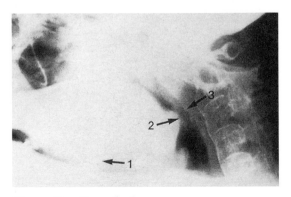

Figure 11 Hyperflexion

Figure 14 Mallampati oropharyngeal scale. Reproduced with permission from Mallanpati SR, Galt SP, Gugino LD, *et al*. A clinical sign to predict difficult intubation: a prospective study. *Can Anaesth Soc* J 1985;32:429–34

class II cases with easy (grade I–III) intubation in 65% and difficult in 35%, while class III oropharyngeal classification correlated with 7% easy (grade I–II), 60% difficult (grade III) and 33% (grade IV) intubations[53,54]. The Mallampati classification and Cormack grading systems when correlated are essentially equivalent, predicting a 10.4% and 11% incidence of difficult intubation, respectively[55].

Other descriptive scales have been validated in small controlled clinical trials. White and Kander[56] suggested that the most important variable correlating with difficulty of intubation was an increase in posterior mandible depth, hindering displacement of soft tissues by the laryngoscope. Additional factors inhibiting displacement of soft tissues by the laryngoscope include an increase in anterior mandible depth, affecting mobility; a reduction of the occiput to cervical vertebra (C_1) distance; a decreased C_1 to C_2 interspinous gap, hindering cervical extension; and reduced temporomandibular joint mobility, restricting oral excursion[56].

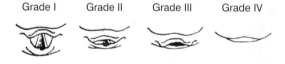

Grade I   Grade II   Grade III   Grade IV

Figure 15 Cormack laryngoscopy scale. Reproduced with permission from Cormack RS, Lehane J. Difficult tracheal intubation in obstetrics. *Anaesthesia* 1984;39:1105–11

Bellhouse and Dore suggested that difficulty with intubation using a curved blade was likely, if there was a failure to visualize the soft palate or uvula, a reduction of one-third of the usual atlanto-occipital extension of 35°, or a recessed chin (2.5 cm anterior to the line of vision)[57]. They documented a failure rate of 20% if the first or all of the last conditions were present[57]. Samsoon and Young compared the failed intubation rate in obstetric patients of 1 in 280 with the rate in general surgical cases of 1 in 2230, documenting a ten-fold increase in incidence[58]. Their retrospective analysis of the intubation failures found that essentially all were cases of Mallampati classification III and Cormack grade IV[58].

Cormack and Lehane reported that grade III and IV patient encounters should occur for every 1 in 2000 or 1 in 10 000 intubations or a single case every 2 or 10 years, respectively[54]. They also suggested a 'blind intubation' technique using the anatomic relationship of the anterior midline epiglottis, lateral piriform sinus and posterior esophagus to advance the stylet and tube into proper position in cases with poor visualization of the glottis[54].

Wilson and associates demonstrated, in a large prospective trial of 633 patients, that the use of posterior laryngeal pressure improved visualization of all but the most severe (grade IV) patients[59]. The rate of failed intubation was reduced significantly from 5.9% to 1.5% with controlled laryngeal pressure[56]. Wilson and colleagues also developed a graded (0,

Table 2 Assessment of intubation difficulty[52–54]

		Cormack laryngoscopy grade			
		1	*2*	*3*	*4*
Visible structures		glottis	posterior glottis	epiglottis	none
Incidence of visualization		99%	1%	1/2000	1/10 000
Mallampati oropharyngeal classification ($n = 210$)					
Visible structures					
I Soft palate	(74%; $n = 155$)	59%	14%	0%	0%
Facial pillars					
Uvula					
II Soft palate	(19%; $n = 40$)	6%	7%	5%	2%
Facial pillars					
III Soft palate	(7%; $n = 15$)	0%	1%	4%	2%
IV None					

least, to 2, most) risk-factor scale citing excess body weight ($p < 0.05$), neck movement ($p < 0.001$), jaw mobility ($p < 0.001$), receding mandible and an overbite, with the former factors correlating independently with difficult intubation[59]. The Predictive Index used rank sum analysis, in which a score of 4 or greater was associated with a false-positive rate of <1% for predicting difficult intubation, but a sensitivity or true-positive rate of only 42% for difficult intubation[59].

Frerk[60] suggested, with use of a preoperative testing strategy developed in 244 patients and using a modified Mallampati scale, that failure of visualization of the posterior pharynx and a thyromental distance of less than 7 cm from chin to thyroid cartilage was associated with difficult intubation. Pottecher and associates[61] evaluated difficult intubation in 663 women, and added to the Mallampati scale, yielding a sensitivity of 84% and specificity of 66%, by examining additional variables, such as mouth opening, chin to hyoid distance, chin to thyroid cartilage distance, dental or facial abnormality, age and weight. The addition of mouth opening to the Mallampati scale improved the accuracy, whereas correlation of dental or facial abnormalities had a mixed effect, increasing the sensitivity but decreasing the specificity.

More general clinical scales have confirmed that the ability to intubate is correlated with the preoperative ability to visualize the oropharynx, as well as with physical examination clues, such as the presence of a short neck, which is strongly associated with the likelihood of a difficult airway[62,63]. Recently, Charters[64] developed a mathematical model for osseous structural factors relating to difficult intubation quantified as the 'inevitable residual volume' of the tongue or the portion remaining anterior to the blade during laryngoscopy. This model uses the tip of the upper incisors, the point on the anterior airway above the larynx, the midpoint between the mandibular condyles and the symphysis midpoint expressed as an F-factor inversely proportional to likelihood of difficult intubation. Lewis and co-workers[65] attempted to produce a clearer definition of the degree of visibility of oropharyngeal structures (OP class) and mandibular space (MS) length. This was accomplished by measurement during different positions of the body, head and tongue and during phonation. The Performance Index was equivalent to $2.5 \times OP$ class – MS length, and ranged from 0 to 2 cm, with a 3.5–24% incidence of difficult intubation[65].

MANAGEMENT STRATEGIES

Effective management strategies for the difficult intubation should involve advance planning with contingency plans for obtaining additional expertise, capability of using alternative techniques or apparatus, and the rapid availability of surgical airway expertise. Difficult-airway algorithms have been developed as a framework for an individualized approach (Figure 16)[66–68]. *Practice Guidelines for Management of the Difficult Airway*, published by the American Society of Anesthesiologists Task Force in 1993, is the current standard of recommendations[69]. The key to avoiding disaster is adequate preparation for the infrequent but inevitable failure to intubate, accompanied by failure to ventilate using rehearsed alternative intubation techniques of the practitioner's choice.

Laryngoscope

The usual response to failed intubation is a change of laryngoscope blade, which has variable results, perhaps less significant for the experienced operator than the novice. Eldor has suggested that blade length and not design may be the crucial element for the novice practitioner[70]. Modification of this strategy recommends the use of a MacIntosh 4 blade, which provides dual capability, allowing either direct or indirect action (Figures 17 and 18).

The more experienced practitioner may choose from an array of blade designs: straight, curved or tubular; handle angle 90°, < 90° or > 90°; and handle configurations. Modern blade development began with Miller, who

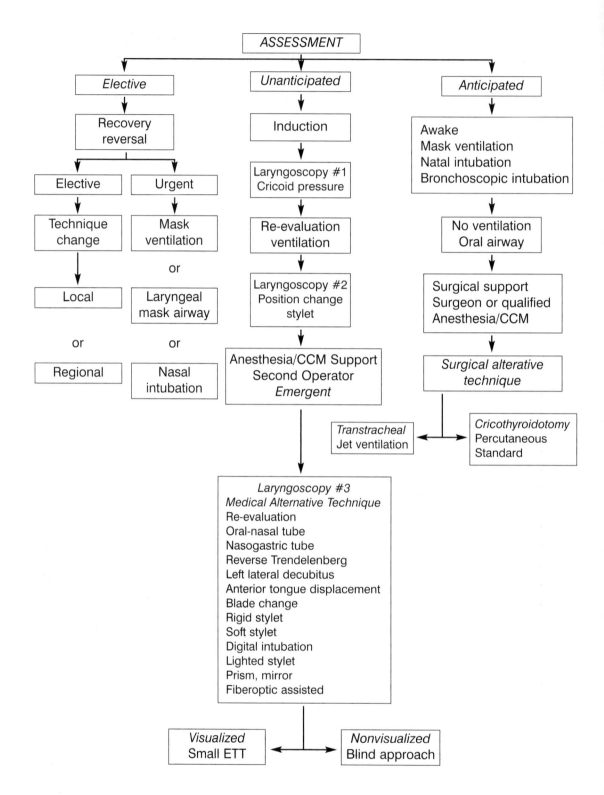

Figure 16 Management strategies for the difficult airway[66–68]

Table 3 Historic development of the laryngoscope

Year	Discoverer	Reference	Type
1827	d'Etoille	5	double blade
1913	Jackson	4	straight U-shaped blade
1941	Miller	6	straight curved tip
1943	MacIntosh	7	curved blade
1944	Flagg	1	straight elevated tip
1944	Wiggin	72	modified C flange
1944	MacBeth	81	obtuse angle
1947	Soper	75	straight with Z flange
1954	Foregger		polio blade
1956	Siker	85	mirror
1958	Bizarri	83	curved with decreased flange
1962	Snow	74	distal tip curvature
1969	Orr	84	right angle
1971	Huffman	87	prism
1973	Schapira	73	thinner Wisconsin
1973	Phillips	10	straight–curved combination
1977	Kessell	92	increased angle
1981	Bantram		short handle
1981	Todres	79	oxyscope
1984	Jellicoe	94	adaptor – open angle
1987	Bainton	77	tubular
1987	Yentis	95	lateral swivel
1987	Wolf	78	oxygen supplementation
1988	Bellhouse	89	midblade level and prism
1991	Crinquette	80	tubular
1993	Biro	86	MacIntosh with mirror

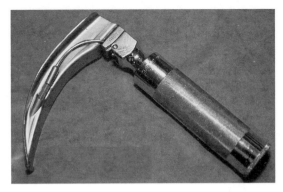

Figure 17 MacIntosh curved blade

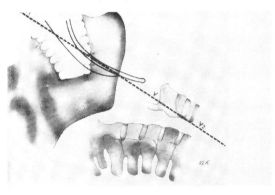

Figure 18 MacIntosh blade indirect line of vision. Reproduced with permission from Phillips OC, Duerksen RL. Endotracheal intubation: a new blade for direct laryngoscopy. *Anesth Analg* 1973;52:691–8

designed a straight thin blade with a distal curve and closed C flange to facilitate ETT passage[6]. The Miller blade, which is longer, allows direct epiglottis contact. The epiglottis has superior laryngeal nerve innervation and is suggested to be more sensitive to stimulation; thus, use of this blade requires a deeper anesthetic state[7] (Figures 19 and 20).

The Flagg blade, a straight design developed in 1944, was later modified by opening the C curvature to increase the protective surface area, decrease the blade angle to 90° and decrease the flange width at the top to facilitate ETT passage[71]. The Wiggin blade incorporates a modified C flange in a similar design[72] (Figure 21).

The Wisconsin blade features a progressive C flange widening towards the distal tip, as opposed to progressive narrowing of the Flagg blade. Also, the inferior flange is shorter than the superior portion of the flange, allowing adequate epiglottis lift and visualization.

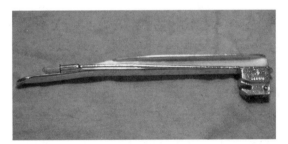

Figure 19 Miller modified straight blade

The Schapira as well as the Whitehead blades are modified Wisconsin designs with decreased flange height, allowing unobstructed vocal cord view if decreased oral excursion or prominent incisors are present[73]. The concave tip design may allow better epiglottis control,

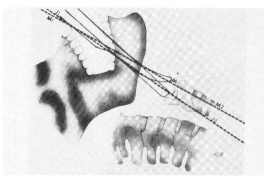

Figure 20 Direct line of vision with the Miller blade. Reproduced with permission from Phillips OC, Duerksen RL. Endotracheal intubation: a new blade for direct laryngoscopy. *Anesth Analg* 1973; 52:691–8

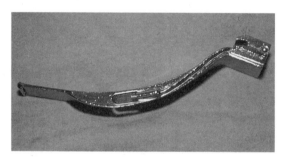

Figure 22 Schapira blade

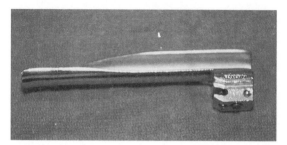

Figure 21 Flagg true straight blade

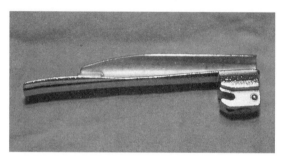

Figure 23 Wisconsin–Foregger straight blade

compensating for a decrease in spatula area (Figure 22).

The Snow blade uses the Wisconsin–Foregger straight blade design modified by a major distal tip curvature instead of the minor curve, as found in the Miller blade[74] (Figure 23).

The Phillips blade is a combination of straight (direct) and curved (indirect) blade characteristics resulting in a straight blade with distal tip curvature, upward illumination and enlarged C flange enabling direct ETT passage. This blade was prospectively evaluated in 1973 by Phillips and Duerksen[10] in 1195 routine operating room patients with anatomic difficulties. The Phillips blade was successful on the first intubation attempt in 84% of cases compared to the Miller (78%), MacIntosh (72%) and Wisconsin–Foregger blades (60%)[10]. Furthermore, the Phillips blade required a stylet in only 17% of cases compared to 20–41% with other straight blades and 66% with a curved blade[10] (Figures 24–26).

The Soper blade combined the straight blade design with the curved-blade Z flange to allow for increased soft tissue displacement to facilitate ETT passage[75].

The Racz–Allen blade is a pressure-sensitive laryngoscope that deforms if excess pressure (> 1.8 kg) is applied to the superior portion of the blade, usually by incisors[76]. Although the blade is protective for dental trauma, it is not particularly adapted to emergency intubation.

The Eversole blade is an early modification of the Jackson straight design with a reduced-sized distal C flange to improve glottic visualization and a 95° handle angle to ease insertion.

The Guedel blade has a 72° handle–blade angle easing insertion, an enlarged C flange acting as a guide for ETT placement and a distal upturned light to increase illumination (Figure 27). The Bennett blade is identical to the Guedel except that the flange has been reduced to facilitate intubation in those patients with decreased oral excursion.

The Mathews blade is a concave spatula design that is introduced into the oropharynx to facilitate passage of a nasotracheal tube.

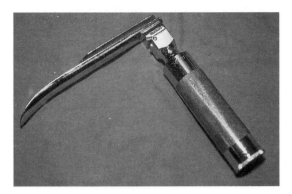

Figure 24   Phillips straight blade

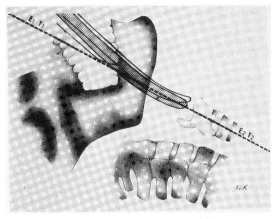

Figure 25   Direct access with enlarged flange (Phillips blade).   Reproduced with permission from Phillips OC, Duerksen RL. Endotracheal intubation: a new blade for direct laryngoscopy. *Anesth Analg* 1973;52:691–8

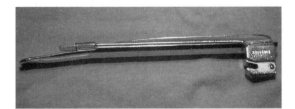

Figure 26   Foregger straight blade

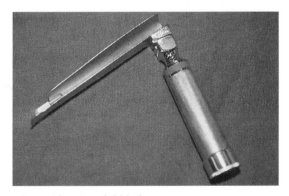

Figure 27   Guedel blade

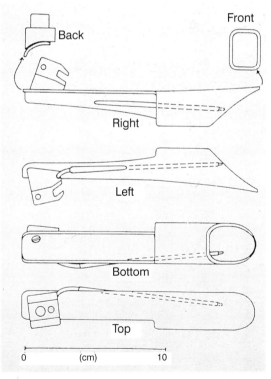

Figure 28   Bainton blade. Reproduced with persmission from Bainton CR. A new laryngoscope blade to overcome pharyngeal obstruction. *Anesthesiology* 1987;67:767–70

Clinical issues such as a decreased oral cavity are addressed by some straight blade designs. Some possess a tubular construction that is effective in providing circumferential displacement for cases of excessive oropharyngeal soft tissue or obstruction. These issues may be addressed with a Bainton blade, a tubular structure with a shielded intraluminal light source for ETT entry through a protected canula[77] (Figure 28). The blade was clinically validated by Bainton in a group of 13 patients with known supraglottic airway obstruction[77]. This tubular laryngoscope design has been modified by Wolf and colleagues to include an oxygen supplementation part for the difficult air-way[78].

The Oxyscope is a straight-blade Miller-type laryngoscope with oxygen supplementation port. Todres and Crone found this device to be associated with a two-fold improvement in arterial oxygenation (43 to 87 mmHg) in a study evaluating neonatal intubation in eight patients with hyaline membrane disease[79].

The Piquet–Crinquette–Vilette (PCV) laryngoscope is an elongated (170 mm) narrow (12 mm) curved device with a tube guide that accepts an 8.0-mm ETT[80]. The PCV device facilitates ETT placement with the device allowed to 'backtrack' over the tube; it has been used successfully in 83% of failed MacIntosh intubations[80].

Pediatric blade design deals with a smaller oropharynx, an enlarged floppy epiglottis and difficulty with neck hyperextension. The Wis–Hipple blade is a straight blade with enlarged C flange and widened distal tip, allowing direct epiglottis contact (Figure 29). The Robertshaw blade has a distal one-third curvature and is designed for indirect epiglottis manipulation. The Seward blade has a uniform even curvature, while the Oxford blade has an acute distal tip angulation with a large flange to combat soft tissue encroachment.

The prototype curved blade design was described by MacIntosh, who suggested that 'this laryngoscope is designed to lessen the difficulty of exposing the larynx to pass an endotracheal tube'[7]. This curved blade is shorter, allowing valleculae contact, has glossopharyngeal innervation and was described as requiring a lighter state of anesthesia for intubation than the Miller blade[7].

The MacIntosh blade with a characteristic reverse Z flange to facilitate visualization has a number of variations (Figure 30). The English MacIntosh features a more acute distal tip angulation, as well as lateral tip offset to improve visualization. The Improved Vision (IV™) MacIntosh (Amtec Medical Products, Sante Fe Springs, CA) establishes a concave surface at the maximal portion of the blade's curvature.

Clinical issues, such as a prominent sternum, are addressed with curved blade designs. MacBeth and Bannister developed an obtuse-handled, open-angled blade, which requires less leverage and is used for conditions of decreased mouth opening or chest prominence[81] (Figure 31). This 'polio blade' further developed by Foregger in 1954 and reported by Weeks[82] is designed with an open angle (123°) configuration (Figure 32). This blade is more effective than straight (90°) or curved (58°) blades avoiding neck flexion in cases of chest prominence, as with a halo cervical fixation device.

The difficulty of intubation in those with decreased oral excursion can be alleviated by the use of the Bizarri–Guffrida blade[83] (Figure 33). This MacIntosh variant eliminates the proximal flange, decreasing the step height to facilitate placement in those with prominent incisors.

Perhaps the most often discussed clinical scenario is the so-called 'anterior larynx'. The Fink blade has an accentuated distally widened tip to improve glottic exposure. The Blechman blade has an even more extreme distal-tip concave angulation to contact positively the

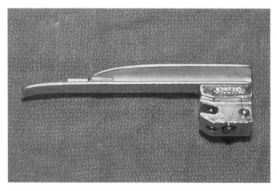

Figure 29 Wis–Hipple pediatric blade

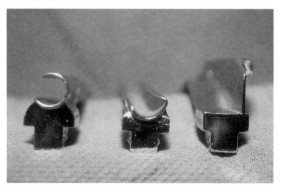

Figure 30 Flange: Z (MacIntosh) vs. C (Miller)

valleculae, deforming the epiglottis with less force.

The Orr blade is also helpful, with an indirect oropharyngeal–laryngeal axis. The blade has a double right-angle bend, which is useful with large incisors or a receding jaw, to avoid a paraxial dental fulcrum[84]. The Choi blade features successive (20°, 30°) angles, culminating in a wide distal tip to improve visualization.

The Siker blade uses a highly polished reflective surface to provide an inverted image, enabling 135° of vision[85]. In a trial of 100 patients, a 99% intubation success rate was reported with the Siker blade with less neck extension, but the inverted image is problematic in an emergency situation[85] (Figure 34). The Biro blade is a modified MacIntosh with a tangential mirror, also utilized successfully in a small clinical trial[86].

The Huffman prism fits on a standard MacIntosh blade to provide line-of-sight viewing with less neck hyperextension and decreased airway tissue deformity[87]. The single-prism version offers an additional 30° of visibility, whereas the double-prism version offers 80° of additional visibility[87] (Figures 35 and 36). This device is better suited to urgent intubation, owing to its right-appearing image[88].

Bellhouse[89] designed a unitized angular (45°) midpoint prism laryngoscope that was used successfully in 3500 intubations, a small portion of which had failed conventional intubation methods. The prism should be maintained at near body temperature to avoid problematic condensation. The Bellscope (International Medical, Burnsville, MN) was studied in a simulated manikin drill using medical student intubators, and was found to be acceptable. However, the standard MacIntosh blade allowed faster, more success-ful tracheal intubations[90].

The McCoy levering laryngoscope features a lever adjacent to the handle, causing forward flexion elevating the epiglottis, improving visualization without excessive force[91].

Additional versatility is offered by consider-ing difficult handle types. Most modifications are directed at the thoracic prominence

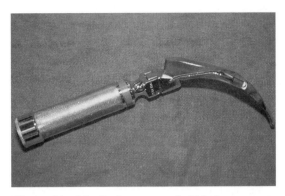

Figure 31   MacBeth open-angled blade

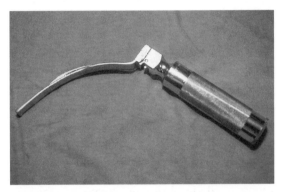

Figure 32   Polio blade – increased angle

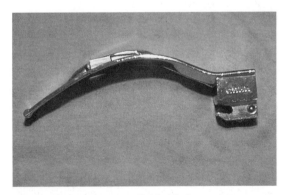

Figure 33   Bizarri–Guffrida blade

clinical scenario encountered in those with polio, pregnancy or a halo fixation device. Modifications required for obstetric intubation increase the blade angle to a more open (110°) configuration to avoid anterior encroachment by a prominent chest[92].

The Bantram handle is a shorter version designed to overcome the thoracic encroachment associated with obesity or pregnancy[93] (Figure 37). However, the mechanical advantage for spatula lift is decreased, requiring more anterior force to be applied. The Howland Lock decreases the angle from 90° to 45° compensating for this decrease in mechanical advantage, improving lift and visualization (Figure 38).

Jellicoe and Harris[94] described an in-line adaptor, and Yentis[95] a lateral swivel adaptor connected to a standard Penlon handle and curved blade that also avoided chest obstruction. The Patil–Syracuse handle is unitized, allowing an adjustment in blade angle from 45° to 180° inversely proportional to mechanical advantage or leverage[96].

The fiberoptic laryngoscope is often utilized as a last-ditch effort in the difficult airway. The Bullard laryngoscope (BLS) (Circon ACMI, Stamford, CT) attempts to approximate conventional design with fiberoptic visualization, offering multiple intubation strategies with and without a stylet in adult and pressor patients[97,98]. The Upsher scope uses the handle with a hollow tube guide, through which the fiberoptic scope is placed with ETT seated for placement.

The Bullard intubating laryngoscope allows a 55° angle of vision complemented by a 90° stylet origination. The vocal cords are visualized, ETT and stylet are placed above the blade, the entire assembly is advanced to the vocal cords, the ETT and stylet are advanced, followed by the blade, and then the stylet is withdrawn[99] (Figures 39 and 40).

However, the Lee Fiberview (Anesthesia Medical Specialties, Santa Fe Springs, CA) laryngoscope adapts a fiberoptic viewing system to a conventional blade design. This device allows for additional 20–30° of visualization, while defaulting to a functional laryngoscope design if required – an optimal design for emergency intubation.

The development and design of the laryngoscope is presented in Table 4[4–8,71–99]. The choice of laryngoscope blade should be modified in accordance with the clinical condition and operator expertise. A classification system based on anatomic variables adapted from MacIntyre is mandatory for the airway expert and desirable for the novice airway practitioner (Table 5)[100]. The recommendations for intubation apparatus are summarized in the difficult-intubation kit (Table 6).

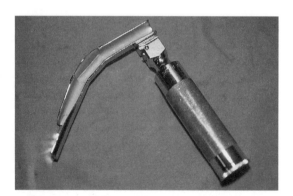

Figure 34 Siker mirror blade

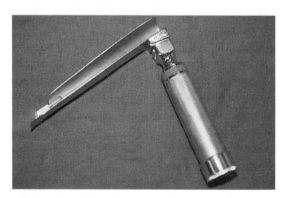

Figure 35 Prism laryngoscope

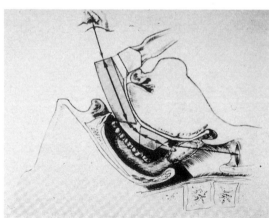

Figure 36 Double prism pharyngolaryngoscope. Reproduced with permission from Huffman JP, Elan JO. Prisms and fiber optics for laryngoscopy. *Anesth Analg* 1971;50:64–7

Stylet

The ETT stylet may be the most important readily available and versatile device in an emergency difficult airway scenario. In 1949, MacIntosh[101] described the use of a soft gum rubber bougie and a malleable stylet for

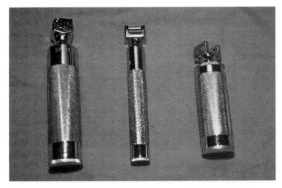

Figure 37 Handle types to increase mechanical advantage regular, thin handle, Bantram handle

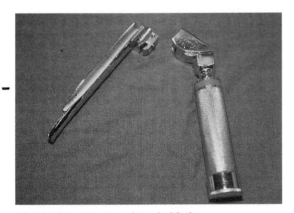

Figure 38 Decreased angle blade

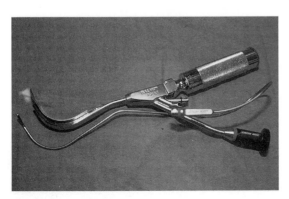

Figure 39 Bullard laryngoscope

assisting intubation. Waters[102] suggested the use of a semi-rigid stylet projecting beyond the ETT and cautious advancement to the trachea in a blind intubation sequence. A potential hazard of the latter technique is tissue damage caused by the stylet. Last, the use of a stylet with an articulated tip allowing acute flexion has been suggested, but is subject to the same 'special instrument' limitations in an emergency situation[103] (Figure 41).

Clinical feasibility trials have confirmed the efficacy of this technique. A malleable stylet and Siker mirror were used successfully in 35 of those who failed conventional intubation attempts[104]. The Flexiguide (Scientific Sales Intl. Inc., Highland Park, IL), a flexible plastic stylet with a directional tip, was 100% successful when used in a series of 17 patients[19]. The Modified Waters' technique of stylet-assisted blind intubation in laryngectomy patients was successful on the first attempt in 31 of 35

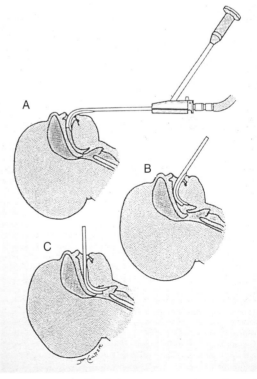

Figure 40 Bullard laryngoscope insertion. **A**, insertion; **B**, oropharynx; **C**, visualization. Stool SE. Intubation techniques of the difficult airway. *Pediatr Infect Dis J* 1988;7:S154–6

Table 4 Anatomic variables and laryngoscope design. From references 4–8, 71–95

Difficulty	Anatomic conditions	Design	Laryngoscope
Prominent sternum	Obesity Poliomyelitis Cast Halo Pregnancy	Increase angle	Polio (128°) MacIntosh (58°), MacBeth (obtuse) Mirror (90°), swivel
Decreased oral excursion	Temporomandibular joint Prominent incision Pierre–Robin syndrome	Decrease flange and step	Schapira (straight) Bizarri–Guffrida (curved) Wisconsin Howland Lock
Reduced oral cavity	Macroglossia Micrognathia Obesity Pregnancy	Increase flange step and surface area	Wisconsin (straight) Flagg Guedel (angle) Bainton Eversole
'Anterior larynx'	Arthritis Cervical injury	Distal tip curvature Moveable tip Angulated Mirror Prism Fiberoptics	Snow (normal) Fink (wide) McCoy Bellhouse Choi Double Angle Siker Biro Huffman Bullard

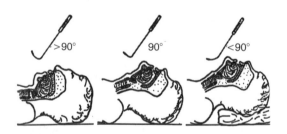

Figure 41 Stylet angle correlated to head position

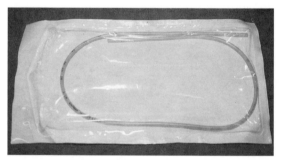

Figure 42 Soft bougie

patients studied by Guggenberger and co-workers[105]. Success occurred on the first intubation attempt in 31 cases and on the second or third in four cases with no complications[105]. A stylet modified to accept jet oxygen flow had a 100% success rate in 59 blind intubation scenarios reported by Bedger and Chang[106].

The soft stylet or bougie has also been used successfully in difficult intubation trials (Figure 42). This device has been found to be the most effective adjunct maneuver, with success in up to one-quarter of failed intubation scenarios[15]. Kidd and colleagues described a blind intubation sequence in 100 simulated and actual difficult (Cormack grade 3) cases resulting in 78% tracheal and 22% esophageal ETT placement[107]. The characteristic tracheal ring bougie tactile contact described as a 'click' is present in 90% of tracheal and absent in 100% of esophageal intubations[107] (Figure 43). The randomized study by Dogra and associates[108] of 100 patients suggested that the proper ETT orientation was bevel posterior (–90°) allowing 100% successful intubations if used initially,

Table 5 Laryngoscope design. From references 4–8, 74–102

Straight
Blade–handle angle 90°
  Jackson: U shape
  Miller: curved tip
  Flagg: narrow C flange
  Wisconsin: wide C flange
  Wisconsin–Foregger: distal open C flange
  Wiggin: modified C flange
  Schapira: decreased flange
  Whitehead: decreased flange
  Snow: major tip curvature
  Phillips: proximal straight, distal curve
  Soper: straight with Z flange
  Racz–Allen–Breakaway
Blade–handle angle >90°
  Eversole
Blade–handle angle <90°
  Guedel: 72°, large C flange
  Bennett: 72°, small C flange

Nasal
Mathews: concave up

Tubular
Bainton: oblong
Wolf: oxygen port
Crinquette: cylindrical

Pediatric
Wis–Hipple: straight
Robertshaw: distal curvature
Seward: uniform curvature
Oxford: acute tip angle

Curved
MacIntosh: uniform curvature
English: offset tip
Low profile, decreased height
MacBeth: obtuse angle
Polio: open angle
Bizarri–Guffrida: decreased flange
Orr: right angle
Choi: double angle
Siker: mirror
Biro: tangential mirror
Huffman: prism adjunct
Bellhouse: angle and prism
McCoy: lever

Handle
Bantram: short handle
Howland: lock-lift adjunct
Jellicoe: open angle adaptor
Yentis: lateral swivel

Fiberoptic
Bullard
Upsher
Lee

Table 6 Difficult-intubation kit

(1)	*Container* Tackle box
(2)	*Airway* Intubating pharyngeal airway (No. 10)
(3)	*Bronchoscopy mask* Laryngeal mask airway (No. 3, 4)
(4)	*Stylette* Lighted
(5)	*Bougie* Tube changer
(6)	*Endotracheal tubes* (a) Micro laryngeal tube – size 5 (b) Reinforced tube
(7)	*Laryngoscope handle* (Incandescent)
(8)	*Laryngoscope blades* (Incandescent) Protruding sternum: adjustable handle Narrow opening Bizzari–Guffrida (No. 4) (c) Excess soft tissue: Guedel (No. 4) (d) Oropharyngeal obstruction: Bainton (Standard) (e) Anterior larynx: Choi (No. 2), McCoy, Blechman, Siker, Huffman Prism
(9)	*Jet ventilator*: catheter (6 Fr) Valve assembly
(10)	*Surgical airway* Percutaneous cricothyroidotomy kit

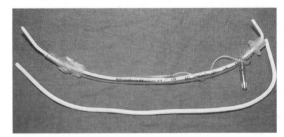

Figure 43 Rigid stylet

and 77% if used to correct a prior unsuccessful attempt. The normal lateral bevel (0°) ETT orientation was successful in only 48% of cases[108].

The Augustine Guide (Augustine Medical Inc., Eden Prairie, MN) uses a plastic guide designed to exit positively in the glottis, allowing passage of a stylet and ETT combination, confirming position with a syringe. The esophageal detector allows free aspiration of tracheal gas while esophageal placement is accompanied by collapse by the suction pressure of -90 cmH$_2$O.

Carr and Belani evaluated the device for the blind endotracheal intubation of 100 patients in neutral head position and were successful in 94% of cases with 71% on first attempt[109]. There were no esophageal intubations, but guide repositioning was required in 23% of cases. Krafft and co-workers reported a success rate of 31 of 33 cases for routine (Mallampati I–II) and seven of eight cases of difficult (Mallampati III–IV) intubation[110]. This device may have utility in those patients in whom glottic visualization (Mallampati IV) is impossible.

Lighted stylet

It is theorized that the posterior ETT orientation allows the bevel to pass along the soft tissue behind the larynx into the trachea. The first lighted stylet was constructed from a malleable stylet and penlight source described by Berman in 1953[111] (Figure 44). The Flexi-Lum® (Concept Corp., Clearwater, FL), composed of a reusable light source and disposable stylet, has been used successfully in operating room trials[112].

In a prehospital study of 21 patients, emergency intubation was 80% successful, with a 67% success rate on the first and 24% success rate on the second intubation attempt[113]. Almost half of the successful intubations occurred after failed conventional attempts, usually within 20 s[113]. However, in a prospective operating room trial of 102 patients, standard laryngoscopy was successful in 98% of first attempts compared to 72% of first attempts with a lighted stylet (Tube-Stat®; Concept Corp., Clearwater, FL), clearly inferior[114] (Figure 45). The lighted stylet was often successful on the second (22%) or third (6%) attempt[114]. Procedural times for the stylet were equivalent (37 to 33 s), with a higher rate of odynophagia (23 to 18%) and

arrhythmia (14 to 2%), but less gagging (26 to 41%) compared to direct laryngoscopy[114].

The lighted stylet has been used successfully as an aid in nasal intubation (Figure 46). Operating room experience suggests a decrease in procedural time (119 to 38 s) and number of attempts (3.1 to 4.1) with epistaxis noted in a stylet-guided compared to a standard nasal intubation approach in a study of 23 patients by Fox and co-workers[115]. The stylet-guided nasal approach was reported in a case of craniofacial dislocation, although it is generally not recommended in such cases[116].

Digital guided intubation

The use of digital guided intubation may be performed blindly or in combination with the lighted stylet[117] (Figure 47). Digital assisted intubation should be performed in only a completely unresponsive or paralyzed patient, although use of a dental prod or bite block has been described in the sedated patient. In this procedure, a bite block is placed, and the middle finger is used to stabilize the epiglottis while the ETT is passed anterior to the curled index finger as a guide to the vocal cords (Figures 48 and 49). The characteristic midline glow at or below the larynx indicates the intertracheal position, whereas a lateral light appearance indicates pyriform sinus malposition, and absent light suggests esophageal malposition (Figures 50 and 51). Emergency medicine service personnel with digital guided intubation found success in 88% of 66 patients, with delay avoided in half of the patients intubated in a study by Hardwick and Bluhm[118].

Nasal intubation

Magill described the first blind nasal intubation performed electively using carbon dioxide as a respiratory stimulant in 1928[119]. Nasal intubation is often the first intubation approach attempted by the novice practitioner, although it requires a significant amount of preparation and skill. The success rate of blind nasal intubation may be as low as 7% in new

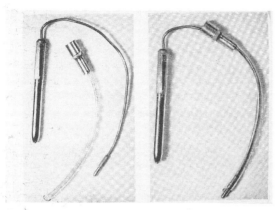

Figure 44   First lighted stylet-penlight adapter

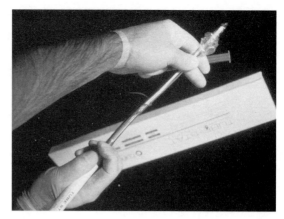

Figure 45   Disposable lighted stylet (Tube-Stat)

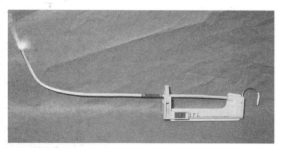

Figure 46   Lighted stylet (STL)

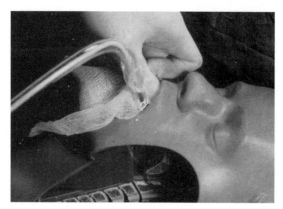

Figure 47   Digital intubation

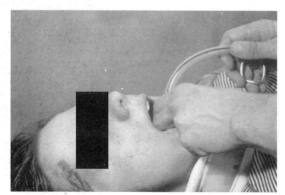

Figure 48   Index finger-guided intubation

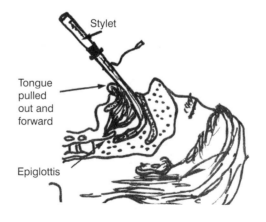

Figure 49   Lighted stylet-assisted digital intubation

trainees[120]. The complications of an improperly performed nasal intubation are significant and include epistaxis, septal hematoma, turbinate disruption, polypectomy or retropharyngeal perforation[121].

Elective nasal intubation with adequate topical vasoconstrictor and local anesthetic enhances both the success rate and the comfort. A modified nasal approach using muscle relaxation increased the nasal intubation success rate to 96% in Fassolt's trial of 52 patients[122], albeit decreasing the margin of safety with failed intubation. Emergency nasotracheal intubation may be less successful (65 to 100%) than succinylcholine-assisted orotracheal intubation. This required increased procedural time (64 to 276 s) without muscle relaxant facilitation in a prospective randomized trial of 52 patients by Dronen and colleagues[123]. The number of attempts was increased (3.7 vs. 1.3) by the nasal route and complications of nasal intubation occurred frequently, including epistaxis (69%), emesis (17%) and aspiration in 1090 of patients[123].

The use of the Beck Airway Flow Monitor (BAAM) (Great Plain Ballistics, Lubbock, TX) assists blind nasotracheal intubation by an audible whistle when near correct tracheal position is achieved; and the Endotrol ETT (Mallinckrodt Critical Care Inc., St Louis, MO), which allows manual guidance to the anterior position, is also helpful[124] (Figure 52). Sloan and Van Rooyen[125] described suction catheter-assisted nasotracheal intubation, where failed attempts require withdrawing the ETT to the oropharynx until the catheter is advanced to the trachea, followed by the ETT. Therefore, nasal intubation can be utilized for emergency intubation in a wide variety of clinical situations.

Awake intubation

Awake intubation is a technique utilizing topical or local anesthesia in an anticipated difficult airway scenario, while the patient usually retains the capability of airway protective reflexes ensuring adequate oxygenation. Thomas[126], in a report of clinical use in an acutely ill population, demonstrated a 100% success rate in all cases with the majority of the 25 patients not experiencing symptoms of discomfort.

The procedure involves local nerve block, specifically the superior laryngeal nerve providing sensation above the vocal cords or the recurrent laryngeal nerve below the vocal cords; topical anesthesia of the oral mucosa, tongue, palate or pharynx; and transtracheal injection through the cricothyroid membrane desensitizing the trachea. All or part of this sequence may be required for adequate airway anesthesia.

This procedure was used by Lee and colleagues[127] in a group of 30 high-risk patients with monitoring of preanesthesia, transtracheal nerve block, and intubation and postintubation periods demonstrating stable blood pressure,

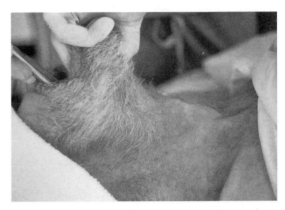

Figure 50 Proper intratracheal position showing midline glow

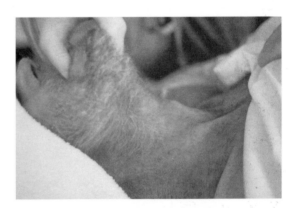

Figure 51 Improper lateral position

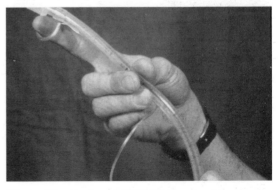

Figure 52 Endotrol ETT (Mallinckrodt)

heart rate and oxygen saturation throughout. Awake intubation may be an acceptable alternative in the urgent intubation situation.

Airway adjuncts

Airway adjuncts include an array of devices providing some degree of airway control. The esophageal obturator airway (Figure 53) was designed for esophageal placement with balloon occlusion and passive gas transfer to the trachea and lungs. However, in clinical practice, two of ten esophageal obturator airway tubes were placed in an intratracheal position (Figure 54) with poor to absent ventilation if unrecognized in a study of ten elective operating room cases reported by Bryson and associates[128]. The esophageal obturator airway is probably not recommended for hospital use, owing to ventilation leak, esophageal trauma, gastric distension or inadvertent obstruction. The limited role remaining for the device is the prehospital environment where the esophageal obturator airway may be used by less experienced personnel. A cuffed nasopharyngeal airway was described by Ralston and Charters[129] as sufficient to maintain ventilation while fiberoptic or other intubation attempts proceeded in a small clinical trial.

The pharyngotracheal lumen airway attempts to achieve the next level of airway control without placement in the trachea itself. This device consists of a 'tube within a tube' consisting of a long esophageal tube with a small balloon and a shorter tracheal tube with a large balloon[130] (Figure 55). Kern and colleagues[131] compared a modified pharyngeal–tracheal airway in a canine arrest model with standard endotracheal intubation and demonstrated an equivalent resuscitation rate. Inadvertent tracheal placement is again an issue and this device has found limited clinical use.

The Combitube (Sheriden, Argyle, NY) tracheal esophageal airway consists of a distal esophageal open-ended tube and proximal tracheal lumen and balloon (Figure 56). The device simplifies proper intraesophageal placement due to its distal opening, but, as in most dual-lumen tubes, proper position is sometimes difficult to verify. The device has been used successfully by Frass and co-workers[132] in a group of 31 cardiac arrest patients providing equivalent oxygenation and ventilation compared to standard endotracheal intubation. This dual-lumen airway is suited to both the prehospital environment and certain in-hospital emergencies.

The logical next development in airway adjunct design is a device that rests immediately superior and apposed to the trachea itself. The Brain Laryngeal Mask was first used in 1985 by Brain in a small group of three operating room patients presenting with an 'anterior larynx'[133] (Figure 57). This device was inserted blindly into the hypopharynx providing adequate oxygenation, while

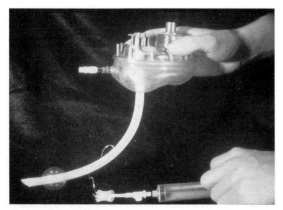

Figure 53 Esophageal obturator device

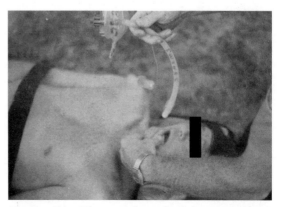

Figure 54 The esophageal obdurator airway inserted

acceptable ventilation was achieved in 15% of the 118 patients evaluated by Brain and colleagues[134].

The device was marketed as the laryngeal mask airway (LMA) and was originally suggested for use for short operative cases (<1 h), supine position and adequate lung mechanics manifested as a continuous positive airway pressure requirement of ≤ 5 cmH$_2$O[135]. However, recent reviews by Brimacombe and co-workers[136] and Asai and Morris[137] illustrate the use of this device in a wide variety of emergency airway scenarios. Verghese and colleagues[138] published their operative experience with 2359 cases, where LMA was used successfully in 99.6% (2350) of patients, with 59% (1399) breathing spontaneously and 41% (960) requiring positive-pressure ventilation. The rate of regurgitation and aspiration was only 0.08%, and no sequelae were encountered in this elective patient group[138]. Also, the device has been placed as an intermediate guide, resulting in a 90% success rate in small (6.0 Fr, 6 mm inner diameter) ETT placement through the central channel of the airway itself[139].

Uncontrolled studies by Silk and colleagues[140] and Kadota and colleagues[141] suggest that placement is achieved utilizing standard and fiberoptic insertion techniques in patients with abnormal airways. Successful LMA positioning has also been achieved in those with neutral head position secondary to a halo device, manual in-line stabilization, cervical spine abnormalities and even prone positioning[142–146].

Clinical reports by Pothmann and associates[16] and Poltronieri[135] suggest successful use of the LMA as an alternative airway, comparing insertion times and correct position in those with cervical collars or decreased neck extension; however, endotracheal intubation more reliably protects patients against

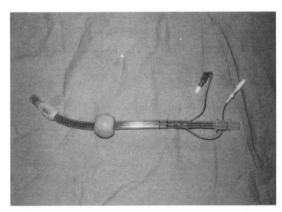

Figure 56 Combitube (Sheriden)

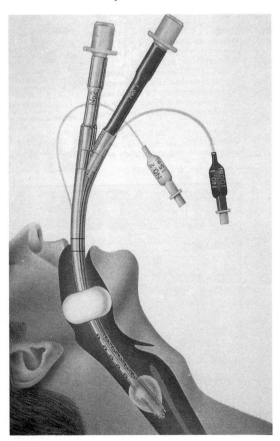

Figure 55 Pharyngotracheal lumen tube

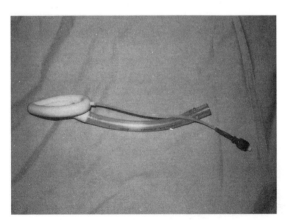

Figure 57 Laryngeal mask airway

aspiration. The device compared favorably to endotracheal intubation in a trial by Reinhart and Simmons[147] of placement by non-physician emergency personnel. There was a greater rate of successful placement with LMA than endotracheal intubation (100% vs. 63%), with fewer attempts (1.0 vs. 2.2) and shorter procedural time (38 vs. 206 s).

Interestingly, the likelihood of successful LMA placement is not predicted by Mallampati or Cormack and Lehane grading scales[148,149]. As clinical experience grows, the LMA has developed into a device that may be used in emergencies instead of elective cases, passed blindly instead of with bronchoscopic guidance, and used for active oxygenation and ventilation continuous positive airway pressure (CPAP ≤ 10–15 cmH_2O) instead of for passive airway control.

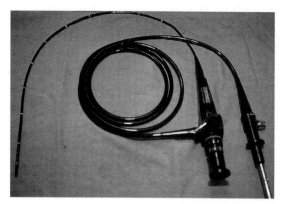

Figure 58   Flexible fiberoptic bronchoscope

Fiberoptic intubation

The fiberoptic laryngoscope is a compact device approximately 35 cm in length and 5.5 mm in width with eyepiece focus and a directional knob to rotate the distal end in a single plane[150] (Figure 58). The device lends itself to the emergency situation with midline insertion and anterior flexion to reach the vocal cords. The intubating laryngoscope is up to 48 cm in length, 3.5–5.5 mm in outer diameter and introduced by an oral route at a 140° angle referenced to 0° for the supine patient compared to the bronchoscope, which is 60 cm in length, 5.9 mm in diameter and introduced by a nasal route requiring a less acute angle of 90–120°[18].

This is best performed as a routine procedure for those with a difficult airway. Fiberoptic intubation is often less successful in the emergency setting. The procedure requires adequate topical anesthesia, with minimal sedation only if required. Adequate ventilation is ensured by a Patil–Syracuse mask offering a bronchoscopic port[151]. Another helpful adjunct is a Berman divided airway allowing quick access to the glottic opening by the oro-pharyngeal route[152]. Proper procedure and practice are essential for this technique to be used for the emergency airway.

The most difficult of airways may some-times be secured by a rigid laryngoscope or bronchoscope. The rigid bronchoscope and ETT are advanced directly to the vocal cords *in situ*[153]. Aro and co-workers[154] discussed a rigid bronchoscopic technique using stylet placement followed by ETT advancement, which was successful in 85% of the 80 patients encountered in the difficult intubation scenario. This scenario occurred at a rate of 2.3% in the 3402 patients analyzed. However, these devices may result in significant complications and should be used only by those personnel skilled in their use, including experts in otolaryn-gology, thoracic surgery or anesthesiology.

The flexible endoscope was first described for nasal intubation in 1967 by Murphy[155]. The flexible fiberoptic bronchoscope has been used successfully in known difficult airway scenarios, such as temporomandibular joint ankylosis or facial abnormalities[156] (Figure 59). The device was 100% successful in a trial of 14 head and neck trauma patients in whom conventional intubation had failed[157]. Hussain[158] studied a similar group of 14 patients, of whom all had an unstable cervical fracture, who underwent oral fiberoptic intubation successfully avoiding a surgical airway. Afilalo and colleagues[159] compared fiberoptic with blind nasotracheal intubation in 42 emergency department patients with an overall success rate of 72% (30) and a range of 56–82% depending on the operator.

Emergency fiberoptic intubation was suc-cessful in 25 of 31 medical patients studied compared to a complete success in four trauma patients studied by Milinek and co-workers[160]. The procedure took slightly longer in the trauma than the medical patients (3 ± 2.2 min vs. 1.8 ± 1.4 min)[160]. Drawbacks include the expense of the device itself; the only failures noted were due to excess secretions or bleeding[160]. An ultrathin pediatric bronchoscope, with a diameter of 2.7 mm compared to the 4.5-mm pediatric and 5.5-mm adult versions, has been used to intubate pediatric patients with Pierre–Robin syndrome and other facial anomalies as described by Kleeman and associates[161].

Emergency bronchoscopic intubation was used by Kalfon and Dubost[162] in 222 cases (Figure 60). It was predominantly performed by the nasal route (98.1%) and was successful in 98.6% of patients usually within 15 min. The failure rate was usually due to excess secretions or bleeding, which were encountered in 17.5% of patients[162]. Another difficulty with fiberoptic intubation is redundant oropharyngeal soft tissue creating a physiological obstruction. Rothfleisch and co-workers[163] described the use of nasal CPAP to 20 cmH$_2$O to the contralateral nares to minimize hypopharyngeal collapse and facilitate translaryngeal bronchoscope passage. Again, maintaining the optic device at near patient body temperature avoids lens condensation.

Retrograde intubation

An early retrograde intubation was reported by Butler and Cirillo in 1960[164]. It was performed through a tracheostomy site using a retrograde stylet and antegrade ETT. The procedure involves a cricothyroid puncture (Figures 61 and 62) entering in a cephalad direction, avoiding the posterior tracheal wall, aspirating air to confirm intratracheal position, advancing a Seldinger wire (20-gauge or 0.021 mm, 18-gauge or 0.035 mm) until oral exit, advancing the stylet or ETT directly until the laryngeal wall contact is noted, advancing the ETT below the vocal cords, and then removing the wire and stylet[165].

This procedure may be adapted to the nasal intubation route by the addition of a nasal to oral wire that is united with the transtracheal to oral wire allowing ETT placement, as reported by Kubo and co-workers[166] in patients with oral neoplasm prior to elective resection. Retrograde

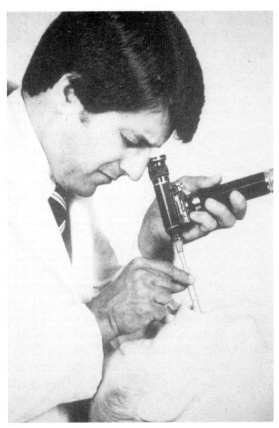

Figure 59 Semi-rigid fiberoptic device

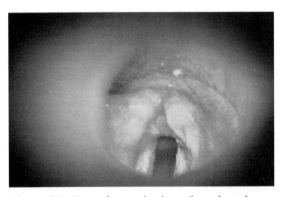

Figure 60 Bronchoscopic view of vocal cords

intubation has been used for emergency cases of maxillofacial trauma and cervical injury. The standard oral intubation was successful in only 68% of 19 trauma patients after 6 ± 1 attempts requiring 18 ± 1 min, whereas the average typical retrograde intubation succeeded in all patients in a single attempt lasting 5 min or less[167].

An additional technical consideration involves the wire exit position from the ETT for proper intratracheal placement. Lleu and colleagues[168] conducted a cadaver study of 77 cases and demonstrated that passage of the wire through the lateral (Murphy) eye of the ETT more often (100%) resulted in the infracricoid position, compared to the distal opening exit site, which was successful in only 29% remaining at the cricothyroid level or above. However, this procedure requires extensive skill to avoid a failed airway or hemorrhage.

Percutaneous jet ventilation

An early jet ventilation procedure was described by Jacoby and colleagues in 1956; a case of complete respiratory obstruction was remedied by an 18-gauge catheter placed through the cricothyroid membrane connected to a low-flow (4 l/min) oxygen system[169].

Initial work by Lassa and associates[170] attempted to increase the cannula size (10-gauge) and to add an exhaust port (Y-connector) to increase flow and ventilation[170]. However, effectiveness was improved by the higher flow rate achieved under a pressurized delivery system (50 psi) available through a standard oxygen wall outlet (Figure 63).

Effectiveness of ventilation is assured by monitoring adequate gas flow controlled predominantly by the pressure gradient. Prophylactic placement of a transtracheal catheter produced acceptable minute ventilation (7.2 l/min) based on conventional jet ventilation settings in clinical use in a study by McLellan and co-workers[171]. Swartzman and associates[172] used a canine model to suggest that percutaneous tracheal jet ventilation (20/min) achieves adequate oxygenation

compared to high-frequency jet ventilation (60/min), although it is prone to some mechanical dysfunction (Figures 64 and 65). In clinical use of percutaneous jet ventilation for elective intubation of eight difficult airway patients, no adverse hemodynamic effects were measured in the cardiac index or ejection fraction[173]. Respiratory needs were met as both oxygenation (arterial oxygen tension 85–240 mmHg) and ventilation

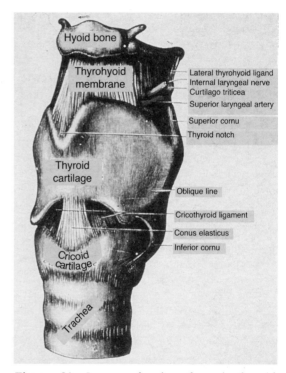

Figure 61 Larynx showing the cricothyroid membrane

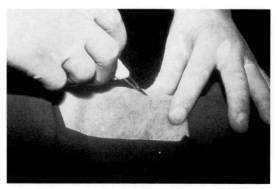

Figure 62 Skin incision

(carbon dioxide tension, 39–44 mmHg) were within acceptable limits[173].

The percutaneous transtracheal jet ventilation strategy has proven effective as a temporizing measure in the difficult airway scenario to ensure adequate oxygenation and ventilation. Weymuller and colleagues[174] reported catheter kinking, lack of respiratory co-ordination, outflow obstruction, excessive secretions or hemorrhage with the device in a study of 13 patients.

However, the most significant risk is catheter obstruction or malposition resulting in gas flow delivered to a closed space, causing tension pneumothorax or subcutaneous emphysema, making further airway efforts and ventilation nearly impossible (Figures 66 and 67). The key is positive confirmation of catheter placement, and manual stabilization to prevent debridement until more conventional airway access can be achieved.

Cricothyroidotomy

Cricothyroidotomy is the prototype emergency surgical airway technique (Figures 68 and 69). This easily performed procedure requires laryngeal cartilage stabilization with cricothyroid membrane identification, vertical skin incision for maximal exposure, horizontal transcricoid stab incision and scalpel replacement with dilator replacement with airway. Perhaps the greatest difficulty related to the procedure is delay in consideration and implementation.

Cricothyroidotomy was revived, owing to the classic review by Brantigan and Grow[175] of the procedure, originally described by Jackson[176], which noted a 61% complication and 0.15% mortality rate. The long-term complication ratio is minor compared to the immediate and ominous implications of a failed airway.

The incidence of failed airway requiring surgical intervention was as high as 7.6% in the review by Esses and Jafek[177] of 1000 patients with an associated mortality rate of 41% and a 2.1% delayed complication rate based on the underlying disease and not the procedure itself. The retrospective review by Spaite and Joseph[178] of 20 prehospital patients defined the indications for a surgical airway as facial trauma in ten (50%), failed oral intubation in nine (45%) and cervical injury in one (5%). The procedure, specifically the skin incision, was anatomically correct in most (94%) cases, but was associated with a 31% complication

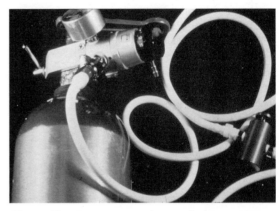

Figure 63   Percutaneous jet ventilation system

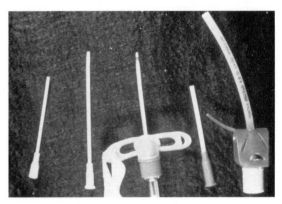

Figure 64   Jet ventilation catheters

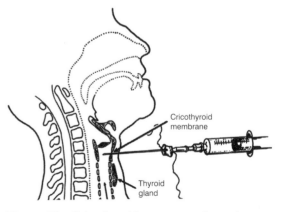

Figure 65   Cricothyroid puncture schematic

Cricothyroid membrane

Thyroid gland

rate. Again, this was a critically ill patient population with an 85% mortality rate and only 5% of survivors returning to their normal state of health[178]. Thus, prehospital cricothyroidotomy is usually performed late in the course in the severely injured, often with little chance of recovery.

However, the use of emergency cricothyroidotomy in expert hands executed at the proper time in the resuscitation period is a potentially life-saving intervention.

CONCLUSION

The approach to the emergency medical airway is best guided by a statement attributed to Gray: 'using an unfamiliar method in an emergency is a recipe for disaster'[54]. The most commonly used intervention in the difficult intubation setting is an alternative laryngoscope blade, stylet, or fiberoptic assistance with concurrent preparation for surgical airway cricothyroidotomy, by either the percutaneous or the open technique (Figures 70–73).

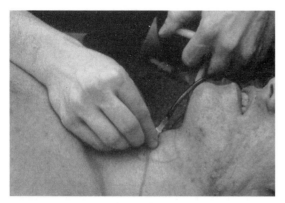

Figure 66 Maintainance of catheter position

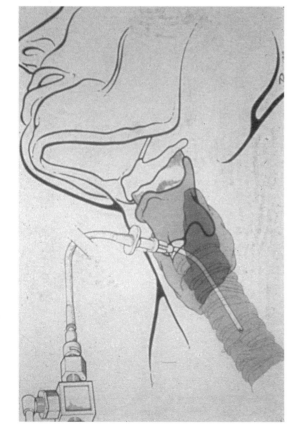

Figure 67 Prevention of kinking that would obstruct gas flow

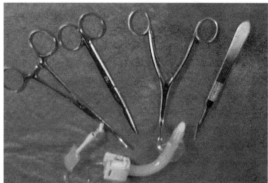

Figure 68 Instruments for use during cricothyroidotomy

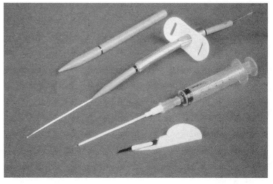

Figure 69 The cricothyroidotomy catheter (Cook)

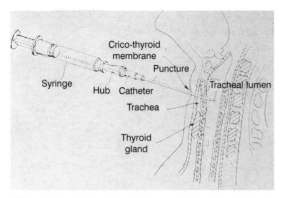

Figure 70   Cricothyroid puncture

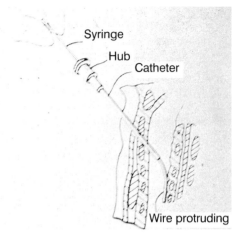

Figure 71   Angle caudad away from posterior wall

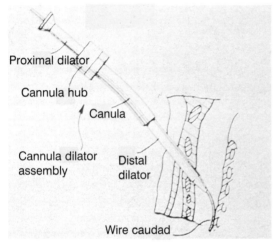

Figure 72   Dilator placement

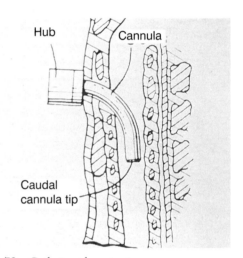

Figure 73   Catheter placement

It would seem that every airway practitioner will encounter at least one difficult intubation, for which a standardized rehearsed algorithm should be implemented based on the operator's expertise.

References

1. Flagg PJ. Introduction. In Flagg PJ, ed. *The Art of Anaesthesia*. Philadelphia: JB Lippincott, 1944:1
2. MacEwen W. Clinical observations on the introduction of tracheal tubes by the mouth instead of performing tracheotomy or laryngotomy. *Br Med J* 1880;2:122–4
3. Jackson C. Instruments. In Jackson C, ed. *Tracheo-Bronchoscopy, Esophagoscopy and Gastroscopy*. St. Louis: St. Louis Laryngoscope Company, 1907:13–62
4. Jackson C. The technique of insertion of intratracheal insufflation tubes. *Surg Gynecol Obstet* 1913;17:507–9

5. d'Etoille L. Recherches sur l'asphyxie. *J Phys* 1827. In Huston KG, ed. *Resuscitation: a Historical Perspective.* Park Ridge, IL: Wood Library-Museum, 1976:31

6. Miller RA. A new laryngoscope. *Anesthesiology* 1941;2:317–20

7. MacIntosh RR. A new laryngoscope. *Lancet* 1943;13:205

8. Stewart RD, Paris PM, Winter PM, *et al.* Field endotracheal intubation by paramedical personnel: success rates and complications. *Chest* 1984;85:341–5

9. Gabram SG, Jacobs LM, Schwartz RJ, *et al.* Airway intubation in injured patients at the scene of an accident. *Conn Med* 1989;53:633–7

10. Phillips OC, Duerksen RL. Endotracheal intubation: a new blade for direct laryngoscopy. *Anesth Analg* 1973;52:691–8

11. Jackson C. Acquiring skill. In Jackson C, ed. *Bronchoscopy and Esophagoscopy: A Manual of Peroral Endoscopy and Laryngeal Surgery.* Philadelphia: WB Saunders, 1922:117–18

12. Stewart RD, Paris PM, Pelton GH, *et al.* Effect of varied training techniques on field endotracheal intubation success rates. *Ann Emerg Med* 1984;13:69–73

13. Goldberg JS, Bernard AC, Marks RJ, *et al.* Simulation technique for difficult intubation: teaching tool or new hazard? *J Clin Anesth* 1990;2:21–6

14. Norton ML, Brown ACD. Evaluating the patient with a difficult airway for anesthesia. *Otolaryngol Clin North Am* 1990;23:771–85

15. Williamson JA, Webb RK, Szekely S, *et al.* The Australian Incident Monitoring Study. Difficult intubation: an analysis of 2000 incident reports. *Anaesth Intensive Care* 1993;21:602–7

16. Pothmann W, Eckert S, Fllekrug B. Use of the laryngeal mask in difficult intubation [German]. *Anaesthetist* 1993;42:644–7

17. Salem MR, Mathrubhutham M, Bennett EJ. Current concepts: difficult intubation. *Med Intell* 1976;295:879–81

18. Edens ET, Sia RL. Flexible fiberoptic endoscopy in difficult intubations. *Ann Otol* 1981;90:307–9

19. Rao TLK, Mathru M, Gorski DW, *et al.* Experience with a new intubation guide for difficult tracheal intubation. *Crit Care Med* 1982;10:882–3

20. Cheney FW, Posner KL, Caplan RA. Adverse respiratory events infrequently leading to malpractice suits. *Anesthesiology* 1991;75:932–9

21. Utting JE, Gray TC, Shelley FC. Human misadventure in anaesthesia. *Can Anaesth Soc J* 1979;26:472–8

22. Craig J, Wilson ME. A survey of anaesthetic misadventures. *Anaesthesia* 1981;36:933–6

23. Beinlich I. Anesthesia-related morbidity and mortality [German]. *Anasthesiol Intensivmed Notfallmed Schmerzther* 1991;26:177–85

24. Lyons G. Failed intubation: six years' experience in a teaching maternity unit. *Anaesthesia* 1985;40:759–62

25. Jay SJ, Johanson WG Jr, Pierce AK. Respiratory complications of overdose with sedative drugs. *Am Rev Respir Dis* 1975;112:591–8

26. Jouppila R, Jouppila P, Hollmen A. Laryngeal oedema as an obstetric anaesthesia complication: case reports. *Acta Anaesth Scand* 1980;24:97–8

27. Suderman VS, Crosby ET, Lui A. Elective oral tracheal intubation in cervical spine-injured adults. *Can J Anaesth* 1991;38:785–9

28. Marcano G, Rabanal JM, Monslera R, *et al.* Subcutaneous emphysema without pneumothorax after difficult intubation [Letter] [Spanish]. *Rev Esp Anestesiol Reanim* 1993;40:319–20

29. Larson SM, Parks DH. Managing the difficult airway in patients with burns of the head and neck. *J Burn Care Rehab* 1988;9:55–6

30. Levitt MWD, Collison JM. Difficult endotracheal intubation in a patient with pseudoxanthoma elasticum. *Anaesth Intensive Care* 1982;5:62–4

31. Drenger B, Zidenbaum M, Reifen E, *et al.* Severe upper airway obstruction and difficult intubation in cicatricial pemphigoid. *Anaesthesia* 1986;41:1029–31

32. Walker RW, Darowski M, Morris P, *et al.* Anaesthesia and mucopolysaccharidosis. A review of airway problems in children. *Anaesthesia* 1994;49:1078–84

33. Walls RD, Timmis DP, Finucane BT. Difficult intubation associated with calcified stylohyoid ligament. *Anaesth Intensive Care* 1990;18:110–26

34. Akinyemi OO, Elegbe EO. Difficult laryngoscopy and tracheal intubation due to calcified stylohyoid ligaments. *Can Anaesth Soc J* 1981;28:80–1

35. O'Sullivan JC, Wells DG, Wells GR. Difficult airway management with neck swelling after carotid endarterectomy. *Anaesth Intensive Care* 1986;4:460–4

36. Potgieter PD, Hammond JMJ. 'Cuff' test for safe extubation following laryngeal edema. *Crit Care Med* 1988;16:818–19

37. Fisher M, Raper RF. The cuff-leak test for extubation. *Anaesthesia* 1992;47:10–12

38. Heindel DJ. Deep neck abscesses in adults: management of a difficult airway. *Anesth Analg* 1987;66:774–6

39. Brahams D. A difficult tracheal intubation as a result of obesity and absence of teeth. *Anaesthesia* 1990;45:586–7

40. Coonan TJ, Hope CE, Howes WJ, *et al.* Ankylosis of the temporo-mandibular joint after temporal craniotomy: a cause of difficult intubation. *Can Anaesth Soc J* 1985;32:158–60

41. Capistrano-Baruh E, Wenig B, Steinberg L, *et al.* Laryngeal web: a cause of difficult endotracheal intubation. *Anesthesiology* 1982;57:123–5

42. Farrell RW, McKenna DM, Breen D, *et al.* A difficult intubation – fatal respiratory arrest secondary to an oral epulis. *J Laryngol Otol* 1992;106:444–5

43. Handler SD, Keon TP. Difficult laryngoscopy/intubation: the child with mandibular hypoplasia. *Ann Otol Rhinol Laryngol* 1983;92:401–4

44. Maydew RP, Berry FA. Cherubism with difficult laryngoscopy and tracheal intubation. *Anesthesiology* 1985;62:810–12

45. Salzarulo HH, Taylor LA. Diabetic 'stiff joint syndrome' as a cause of difficult endotracheal intubation. *Anesthesiology* 1986;64:366–8

46. Edge WG, Whitwam JG. Chondro-calcinosis and difficult intubation in acromegaly. *Anaesthesia* 1981;36:677–80

47. Lee HC, Andree RA. Cervical spondylosis and difficult intubation. *Anesth Analg* 1979;58:434–5

48. Crosby ET, Grahovac S. Diffuse idiopathic skeletal hyperostosis: an unusual cause of difficult intubation. *Can J Anaesth* 1993;40:54–8

49. Cass NM, James NR, Lines V. Difficult direct laryngoscopy complicating intubation for anaesthesia. *Br Med J* 1956;1:488–9

50. Kamath SK, Randive SB, Bhatt MM. Difficult intubation – when can we predict it? *J Postgrad Med* 1991;37:40–3

51. Hotchkiss RS, Hall JR, Braun IF, *et al.* An abnormal epiglottis as a cause of difficult intubation – airway assessment using magnetic resonance imaging. *Anesthesiology* 1988;68:140–2

52. Mallampati SR. Clinical sign to predict difficult tracheal intubation (hypothesis). *Can Anaesth Soc J* 1983;30:316–17

53. Mallampati SR, Gugino LD, Desai SP, *et al.* A clinical sign to predict difficult tracheal intubation: a prospective study. *Can Anaesth Soc J* 1985;32:429–34

54. Cormack RS, Lehane J. Difficult tracheal intubation in obstetrics. *Anaesthesia* 1984;39:1105–11

55. Restelli L, Moretti MP, Todaro C, *et al.* The Mallampati's scale: a study of reliability in clinical practice [Italian]. *Minerva Anestesiol* 1993;59:261–5

56. White A, Kander PL. Anatomical factors in difficult direct laryngoscopy. *Br J Anaesth* 1975;47:468–74

57. Bellhouse CP, Dore C. Criteria for estimating likelihood of difficulty of endotracheal intubation with the MacIntosh laryngoscope. *Anaesth Intensive Care* 1988;16:329–37

58. Samsoon GLT, Young JRB. Difficult tracheal intubation: a retrospective study. *Anaesthesia* 1987;42:487–90

59. Wilson ME, Spiegelhalter D, Robertson JA, *et al*. Predicting difficult intubation. *Br J Anaesth* 1988;61:211–16

60. Frerk CM. Predicting difficult intubation. *Anaesthesia* 1991;46:1005–8

61. Pottecher T, Velten M, Galani M, *et al.* Comparative value of clinical signs of difficult tracheal intubation in women [French]. *Ann Fr Anesth Reanim* 1991;10:430–5

62. Cohen SM, Laurito CE, Segil LJ. Examination of the hypopharynx predicts ease of laryngoscopic visualization and subsequent intubation: a prospective study of 665 patients. *J Clin Anesth* 1992;4:310–14

63. Rocke DA, Murray WB, Rout CC, *et al.* Relative risk analysis of factors associated with difficult intubation in obstetric anesthesia. *Anesthesiology* 1992;71:67–73

64. Charters P. Analysis of mathematical model for osseous factors in difficult intubation. *Can J Anaesth* 1994;41:594–602

65. Lewis M, Keramati S, Benumof JL, *et al.* What is the best way to determine oropharyngeal classification and mandibular space length to predict difficult laryngoscopy? *Anesthesiology* 1994;81:69–75

66. Davies JM, Weeks S, Crone LA, *et al.* Difficult intubation in the parturient. *Can J Anaesth* 1989;36:668–74

67. Benumof JL. Management of the difficult adult airway. With special emphasis on awake tracheal intubation. *Anesthesiology* 1991;75:1087–110

68. Schwartz DE, Wiener-Kronish JP. Management of the difficult airway. *Clin Chest Med* 1991;12:483–95

69. ASA Task Force. Practice guidelines for management of the difficult airway. A report by the American Society of Anesthesiologists Task Force on management of the difficult airway. *Anesthesiology* 1993;78:597–602

70. Eldor J. The length of the blade is more important than its design in difficult tracheal intubation. *Can J Anaesth* 1990;37:268

71. Flagg PJ. Intratracheal inhalation anesthesia in practice. *Arch Otolaryngol Head Neck Surg* 1932;15:844–59

72. Wiggin SC. A new modification of the conventional laryngoscope and technique for laryngoscopy. *Anesthesiology* 1944;5:61–8

73. Schapira M. A modified straight laryngoscope blade designed to facilitate endotracheal intubation. *Anesth Analg* 1973;52:553–4

74. Snow JC. Modification of laryngoscope blade. *Anesthesiology* 1962;23:394

75. Soper RL. A new laryngoscope for anesthetists. *Br Med J* 1947;1:265

76. Racz GB, Allen FB. A new pressure-sensitive laryngoscope. *Anesthesiology* 1985;62:356–8

77. Bainton CR. A new laryngoscope blade to overcome pharyngeal obstruction. *Anesthesiology* 1987;67:767–70

78. Wolf C, LeJeune FE Jr, Douglas JR Jr. A technique for intubation of the difficult airway. *Otolaryngol Head Neck Surg* 1987;96:278–81

79. Todres ID, Crone RK. Experience with a modified laryngoscope in sick infants. *Crit Care Med* 1981;9:544–5

80. Crinquette V, Vilette B, Solanet C, *et al.* Use of the PVC, a laryngoscope for difficult intubation [French]. *Ann Fr Anesth Reanim* 1991;10:589–94

81. MacBeth RG, Bannister FB. A new laryngoscope. *Lancet* 1944;247:660

82. Weeks DB. A new use for an old blade. *Anesthesiology* 1974;40:200–1

83. Bizarri DV, Guffrida JG. Improved laryngoscope blade designed for ease of manipulation and reduction of trauma. *Anesth Analg* 1958;37:231–2

84. Orr RB. A new laryngoscope blade designed to facilitate difficult endotracheal intubation. *Anesthesiology* 1969;31:377–8

85. Siker ES. A mirror laryngoscope. *Anesthesiology* 1956;17:38–42

86. Biro P. A modified MacIntosh blade for difficult intubation. The mirror blade [German]. *Anaesthetist* 1993;42:105–10

87. Huffman JP, Elam JO. Prisms and fiberoptics for laryngoscopy. *Anesth Analg* 1971;50:64–7

88. Huffman JP. An indirect–direct laryngoscope. *Anesth Analg* 1975;54:404

89. Bellhouse CP. An angulated laryngoscope for routine and difficult tracheal intubation. *Anesthesiology* 1988;69:126–9

90. Hodges UM, O'Flaherty D, Adams AP. Tracheal intubation in a manikin: comparison of the Bellscope with the MacIntosh laryngoscope. *Br J Anaesth* 1993;71:905–7

91. McCoy EP, Mirakhur RK. The levering laryngoscope. *Anesthesia* 1993;48:516–19

92. Kessell J. A laryngoscope for obstetrical use an obstetrical laryngoscope. *Anaesth Intensive Care* 1977;5:265–6

93. Datta S. Modified laryngoscope for endotracheal intubation of obese patients. *Anesth Analg* 1981;60:120–1

94. Jellicoe JA, Harris NR. A modification of a standard laryngoscope for difficult tracheal intubation in obstetric cases. *Anaesthesia* 1984;39:800–2

95. Yentis SM. A laryngoscope adaptor for difficult intubation. *Anaesthesia* 1987;42:764–6

96. Patil VU, Stehling LC, Zauder HL. An adjustable laryngoscope handle for difficult intubations. *Anesthesiology* 1984;60:609

97. Saunders PR, Geisecke AH. Clinical assessment of the adult Bullard laryngoscope. *Can J Anaesth* 1989;36:S118–S119

98. Stool SE. Intubation techniques of the difficult airway. *Pediatr Infect Dis J* 1988;7:S154–S156

99. Riou B, Langeron O, Fabas E, *et al.* Intratracheal intubation using a fiberoptic laryngoscope [French]. *Ann Fr Anesth Reanim* 1991;10:308–10

100. McIntyre JWR. Laryngoscope design and the difficult adult tracheal intubation. *Can J Anaesth* 1989;36:94–8

101. MacIntosh RR. An aid to oral intubation. *Br Med J* 1949;1:28

102. Waters DI. Guided blind retrograde intubation: for patients with deformities of the upper airway. *Anaesthesia* 1963;18:158–62

103. Henderson JB, Bontrager E, Morse HT. An articulated stylet for endotracheal intubation. *Anesthesiology* 1970;32:71–3

104. Tahir AH, Renegar OJ. A stylet for difficult orotracheal intubation. *Anesthesiology* 1973;39:337–9

105. Guggenberger H, Lenz G, Heumann H. Erfolgsrate und Komplikationen einer modifizierten retrograden intubationstechnik bei 36 patienten. *Anaesthetist* 1987;36:703–7

106. Bedger RC Jr, Chang JL. A jet-stylet endotracheal catheter for difficult airway management. *Anesthesiology* 1987;66:221–3

107. Kidd JF, Dyson A, Latto IP. Successful difficult intubation: use of the gum elastic bougie. *Anaesthesia* 1988;43:437–8

108. Dogra S, Falconer R, Latto IP. Successful difficult intubation: tracheal tube placement over a gum-elastic bougie. *Anaesthesia* 1990;45:774–6

109. Carr RJ, Belani KG. Clinical assessment of the Augustine Guide for endotracheal intubation. *Anesth Analg* 1994;78:983–7

110. Krafft P, Fitzgerald R, Pernerstorefer T, *et al.* A new device for blind oral intubation in routine and difficult airway management. *Eur J Anesthesiol* 1994;11:207–12

111. Berman RA. Lighted stylet. *Anesthesiology* 1959;20:282–3

112. Ducrow M. Throwing light on blind intubation. *Anaesthesia* 1978;33:827–9

113. Vollmer TP, Stewart RD, Paris PM, *et al.* Use of a lighted stylet for guided orotracheal intubation in the prehospital setting. *Ann Emerg Med* 1985;14:325–8

114. Ellis DG, Jakymec A, Kaplan RM, *et al.* Guided orotracheal intubation in the operating room using a lighted stylet: a comparison with direct laryngoscopic technique. *Anesthesiology* 1986;64:823–6

115. Fox DJ, Castro T Jr, Rastrelli AJ. Comparison of intubation techniques in the awake patient: the Flexi-Lum surgical light (lightwand) versus blind nasal approach. *Anesthesiology* 1987;66:69–71

116. Verdile VP, Heller MB, Paris PM, *et al.* Nasotracheal intubation in traumatic craniofacial dislocation: use of the lighted stylet. *Am J Emerg Med* 1988;6:39–41

117. Stewart RD. Tactile orotracheal intubation. *Ann Emerg Med* 1984;13:175–8

118. Hardwick WC, Bluhm D. Digital intubation. *J Emerg Med* 1984;1:317–20

119. Magill IW. Endotracheal anaesthesia. *Proc R Soc Med* 1928;22:83

120. McHale SP, Brydon CW, Wood MLB, *et al.* A survey of nasotracheal intubating skills among Advanced Trauma Life Support course graduates. *Br J Anaesth* 1994;72:195–7

121. Gallagher JV, Vance MV, Beechler C. Difficult nasotracheal intubation: a previously unreported anatomical cause. *Ann Emerg Med* 1985;14:258–60

122. Fassolt A. Blind nasotracheal intubation in the muscle-relaxed patient [German]. *Anaesthetist* 1986;35:504–8

123. Dronen SC, Merigian KS, Hedges JR, *et al.* A comparison of blind nasotracheal and succinyl-choline-assisted intubation in the poisoned patient. *Ann Emerg Med* 1987;16:650–2

124. Cook RT Jr, Stene JK Jr. The BAAM and Endotrol endotracheal tube for blind oral intubation. Beck Airway Air Flow Monitor. *J Clin Anesth* 1993;5:431–2

125. Sloan EP, Van Rooyen MJ. Suction catheter-assisted nasotracheal intubation. *Acad Emerg Med* 1994;1:388–90

126. Thomas JL. Awake intubation indications, techniques and review of 25 patients. *Anaesthesia* 1969;24:28–35

127. Lee LS, Chau SW, Yu KL, *et al.* Clinical study of awake fiberoptic nasotracheal intubation for difficult opening mouth patients [Chinese]. *Ma Tsui Hsueh Tsa Chi* 1990;28:343–9

128. Bryson TK, Benumof JL, Ward CF. The esophageal obturator airway: a clinical comparison to ventilation with a mask and oropharyngeal airway. *Chest* 1978;74:537–9

129. Ralston SJ, Charters P. Cuffed naso-pharyngeal tube as 'dedicated airway' in difficult intubation. *Anaesthesia* 1994;49:133–6

130. Bartlett RL, Martin SD, Perina D, *et al.* The pharyngo-tracheal lumen airway: an assessment of airway control in the setting of upper airway hemorrhage. *Ann Emerg Med* 1987;16:343–6

131. Kern K, Nelson J, Norman S, *et al.* Oxygenation and ventilation during cardio-pulmonary resuscitation utilizing continuous oxygen delivery via a modified pharyngeal–tracheal lumen airway. *Chest* 1992;101:522–9

132. Frass M, Frenzer R, Rauscha F, *et al.* Evaluation of esophageal tracheal combitube in cardiopulmonary resuscitation. *Crit Care Med* 1986;15:609–11

133. Brain AIJ. Three cases of difficult intubation overcome by the laryngeal mask airway. *Anaesthesia* 1985;40:353–5

134. Brain AI, McGhee TD, McAteer EJ, *et al.* The laryngeal mask airway. Development and preliminary trials of a new type of airway. *Anaesthesia* 1985;40:356–61

135. Poltronieri J. The laryngeal mask [French]. *Ann Fr Anesth Reanim* 1990;9:362–6

136. Brimacombe J, Berry A, Brain A. The laryngeal mask airway. *Anesthesiol Clin North Am* 1995;13:411–37

137. Asai T, Morris S. The laryngeal mask airway: its features, effects and role. *Can J Anaesth* 1994;41:930–60

138. Verghese C, Smith TGC, Young E. Prospective survey of the use of the laryngeal mask airway in 2359 patients. *Anaesthesia* 1993;48:58–60

139. Heath ML. Endotracheal intubation through the laryngeal mask – helpful when laryngoscopy is difficult or dangerous. *Eur J Anesthesiol* 1991;4(Suppl):41–5

140. Silk JM, Hill HM, Calder I. Difficult intubation and the laryngeal mask. *Eur J Anaesthesiol* 1991;4:47–51

141. Kadota Y, Oda T, Yoshimura N. Application of a laryngeal mask to a fiberoptic bronchoscope-aided tracheal intubation. *J Clin Anesth* 1993;5:226–30

142. Pennant JH, Pace NA, Gajraj NM. Role of the laryngeal mask airway in the immobile cervical spine. *J Clin Anesth* 1993;5:226–30

143. Brimacombe J, Berry A. Laryngeal mask airway insertion. A comparison of the standard versus neutral position in normal patients with a view to its use in cervical spine instability. *Anaesthesia* 1993;48:670–1

144. Logan A. Use of the laryngeal mask in a patient with an unstable fracture of the cervical spine. *Anaesthesia* 1991;46:987

145. Lee JJ, Yau K, Barcroft J. LMA and respiratory arrest after anterior cervical fusion. *Can J Anaesth* 1993;40:395–6

146. Milligan KA. Laryngeal mask in the prone position. *Anaesthesia* 1994;49:449

147. Reinhart D, Simmons G. Comparison of placement of the laryngeal mask airway with endotracheal tube by paramedics and respiratory therapists. *Ann Emerg Med* 1994;24:260–3

148. Brimacombe J, Berry A. Mallampati classification and laryngeal mask insertion. *Anaesthesia* 1993;48:347

149. Mahiou P, Narchi P, Veyrac P, *et al.* Is laryngeal mask easy to use in case of difficult intubation? *Anesthesiology* 1992;77:A1228

150. Witton TH. An introduction to the fiberoptic laryngoscope. *Can Anaesth Soc J* 1981;28:475–8

151. Patil C. Concerning the complications of the Patil–Syracuse mask. *Anesth Analg* 1993;76:1162–78

152. Berman RA. A method for blind oral intubation of the trachea or esophagus. *Anesth Analg* 1977;56:866–7

153. Mirakhur RK. Technique for difficult intubation. *Br J Anaesth* 1972;44:632

154. Aro L, Takki S, Aromaa U. Technique for difficult intubation. *Br J Anaesth* 1971;43:1081–2

155. Murphy P. A fibre-optic endoscope used for nasal intubation. *Anaesthesia* 1967;22:489–91

156. Mishke L, Wang JF, Gutierrez F, *et al.* Nasotracheal intubation by fiberoptic laryngoscope. *South Med J* 1981;74:1407–9

157. Mulder DS, Wallace DH, Woolhouse FM. The use of fiberoptic bronchoscope to facilitate endotracheal intubation following head and neck trauma. *J Trauma* 1975;15:638–40

158. Hussain SA. The fiberoptic bronchoscope. *J Am Coll Emerg Physicians* 1977;6:500–3

159. Afilalo M, Guttman A, Stern E, *et al.* Fiberoptic intubation in the emergency department. *J Emerg Med* 1993;11:387–91

160. Milinek EJ Jr, Clinton JE, Plummer D, *et al.* Fiberoptic intubation in the emergency department. *Ann Emerg Med* 1990;19:359–62

161. Kleeman PP, Jantzen JP, Bonfils P. The ultra-thin bronchoscope in management of the difficult pediatric airway. *Can J Anaesth* 1987;34:606–8

162. Kalfon F, Dubost J. Use of fiberoptic broncho-scope for difficult intubation in maxillofacial surgery [French]. *Ann Fr Anesth Reanim* 1993;12:278–83

163. Rothfleisch R, Davis LL, Kuebel DA, *et al.* Facilitation of fiberoptic nasotracheal intubation in a morbidly obese patient by simultaneous use of nasal CPAP. *Chest* 1994;106:287–8

164. Butler FS, Cirillo AA. Retrograde tracheal intubation. *Anesth Analg (Cleve)* 1960;39:333–8

165. Borland LM, Swan DM, Leff S. Difficult pediatric endotracheal intubation: a new approach to the retrograde technique. *Anesthesiology* 1981;55:577–8

166. Kubo K, Takahashi S, Oka M. A modified technique of guided blind intubation in oral surgery. *J Maxillofac Surg* 1980;8:135–7

167. Barriot P, Riou B. Retrograde technique for tracheal intubation in trauma patients. *Crit Care Med* 1988;16:712–13

168. Lleu JC, Forrler M, Forrler C, *et al.* Retrograde orotracheal intubation [French]. *Ann Fr Anesth Reanim* 1989;8:632–5

169. Jacoby JJ, Harmelbury W, Ziegler CH, *et al.* Transtracheal resuscitation. *J Am Med Assoc* 1956;162:625–8

170. Lassa RE, Habal MB, Ross N, *et al.* Rapid access airway surgical device and technique. *Int Surg* 1978;63:152

171. McLellan I, Gordon P, Khawaja S, *et al.* Percutaneous transtracheal high frequency jet ventilation as an aid to difficult intubation. *Can J Anaesth* 1988;35:404–5

172. Swartzman S, Wilson MA, Hoff BH, *et al.* Percutaneous transtracheal jet ventilation for cardiopulmonary resuscitation: evaluation of a new jet ventilator. *Crit Care Med* 1984;12:8–13

173. Nakatsuka M, MacLeod AD. Hemodynamic and respiratory effects of transtracheal high-frequency jet ventilation during difficult intubation. *J Clin Anesth* 1992;4:321–4

174. Weymuller EA Jr, Pavlin EG, Paugh D, *et al.* Management of difficult airway problems with percutaneous transtracheal ventilation. *Ann Otol Rhinol Laryngol* 1987;96:34–7

175. Brantigan CO, Grow JB Sr. Cricothyroid-otomy: elective use in respirator problems requiring tracheotomy. *J Thorac Cardiovasc Surg* 1976;71:72–81

176. Jackson C. High tracheotomy and other errors the chief causes of chronic laryngeal stenosis. *Surg Gynecol Obstet* 1921;32:392–8

177. Esses BA, Jafek BW. Cricothyroidotomy: a decade of experience in Denver. *Ann Otol Rhinol Laryngol* 1987;96:519–24

178. Spaite DW, Joseph M. Prehospital crico-thyrotomy: an investigation of indications, technique, complications, and patient outcome. *Ann Emerg Med* 1990;19:279–85

Confirmation of endotracheal tube placement 3

INTRODUCTION

Emergency airway control has been described since as early as 3600 BC, when tracheostomy was used by the Egyptians[1]. Modern interventions include the introduction of endotracheal tubes (ETTs) for anesthesia by MacEwen in 1880[2], but the first clinical use of endotracheal intubation for airway control was advanced by Jackson in 1907[3].

Endotracheal intubation is associated with an approximate complication rate of 26%[4]. Perhaps the most catastrophic outcome of this procedure is unrecognized esophageal intubation[5]. Fully 15% of anesthesia-related accidents resulting in brain damage or death are the result of esophageal intubation. This patient care hazard is illustrated by the statement that 'even a conscientious, careful anesthesiologist may be unable to differentiate tracheal from esophageal intubation by commonly employed methods'[6]. Accidental esophageal intubation has been reported in even well-controlled anesthesia settings, as well as in the prehospital realm[7-9], where ineffective airway management may be the most important factor contributing to out-of-hospital deaths[10]. In a study of paramedic intubations of 799 patients, Stewart and colleagues found a 9.5% complication rate, with 1.8% resulting in esophageal misplacement of the endotracheal tube[11].

ETT position is suggested but not confirmed by a number of techniques. The general guidelines for an ideal method[12] are:

(1) The test should work for difficult intubations;

(2) Positive tests must be unequivocal;

(3) Esophageal intubation must always be detected;

(4) Clinicians must understand the test.

CONFIRMATION

Techniques for clinical evaluation of ETT position include direct visualization[8], ventilation-bag compliance[8,13], auscultation of breath sounds[8,13,14], symmetrical chest excursion[13], auscultation of epigastric sounds[8,15], vital sign change[8], cyanosis or hypoxemia[16], tracheal cuff palpation[17-19], tactile digital palpation[20], chest compression[8], flexible fiberoptic catheter bronchoscopy[21,22], suction esophageal detection device[23,24], pulse oximetry[15,25-28], lighted stylet[29], cuff seal volume[30], chest radiograph[31-33], ultrasound[34], exhaled tidal volume[7], tube condensation[8], gastric contents[15], colorimetric end-tidal CO_2 detector[35] and end-tidal CO_2 measurement[15]. Each of these techniques has been suggested to confirm ETT position; although they vary in their accuracy, some conclusions can be inferred from the data (Figures 1–5).

Clinical testing cannot be relied on exclusively, and the only unequivocal signs of correct tube placement are direct visualization, including recheck laryngoscopy, fiberoptic bronchoscopic identification of the endotracheal lumen and detection of a physiological CO_2 concentration in exhaled gas[24]. However, each of these gold standards has been associated with some limitation. Direct visualization may be the most reliable technique, although it is not always anatomically possible[36]. The ETT can be accidentally dislodged, and 1.9 cm of change in ETT position with normal head flexion or extension has been documented in radiographic evaluation[37]. Radiographic assessment has been associated with delayed diagnosis, resulting in prolonged esophageal intubation[31]. Bronchoscopy requires special apparatus and ability, and is time consuming. Pulse oximetry may be limited by a delay in the detection of oxyhemoglobin desaturation, especially with anticipating preoxygenation,

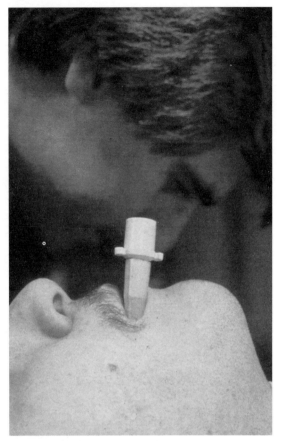

Figure 1 Confirmation of tube placement by auscultation

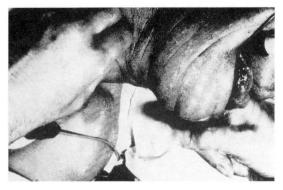

Figure 2 Tracheal cuff palpation

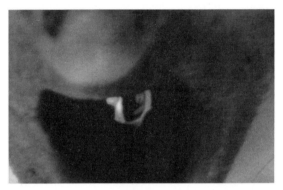

Figure 3 Direct visualization

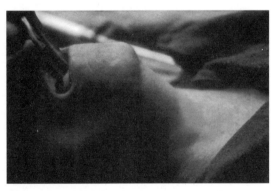

Figure 4 Lighted stylet to assess tube placement

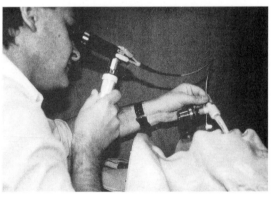

Figure 5 Bronchoscopic visualization of tube placement

as well as by inability to sense CO_2 during a low-flow state[25].

MONITORING

CO_2 monitoring 'comes closest to being a fail-safe monitor for most problems that cause anoxia and death'[38]. The earliest experiments in CO_2 measurement were performed by

Tyndall (1859) and Luft (1943) who developed the principle of capnometry, by which CO_2 is measured by infrared absorption[39]. Primitive attempts at crude CO_2 measurement were made in the anesthesia suite by the barium hydroxide agglutination reaction[40] and the 'Einstein CO_2 detector', which was capable of sensing 4–6 vol% CO_2[41].

Modern CO_2 measurement may be accomplished by two methods. Mass spectroscopy requires a centralized system suited for anesthesia and intensive care settings. Expired gas is sampled and examined for CO_2 as well as other volatile gases. This mode is the current standard. However, this method requires calibration and is costly – about $60 000 for an average system[42]. End-tidal CO_2 measurement is based on the absorption of infrared light of 4.3-pm wavelength by the CO_2 molecule compared with a CO_2-free reference sample[29]. Sampling occurs through a side-stream system, which requires anesthetic gas removal, is prone to contamination, and is used for mass spectroscopy and some capnography. Mainstream detectors place the sensor directly into the airway circuit, offer less contamination and are featured in capnographs and capnometers. A band filter is featured to screen out other anesthetic gases.

The CO_2 concentration can be displayed in either qualitative (with an arbitrary CO_2 sensitivity) or quantitative fashion. Quantitative display includes capnometry, which yields a numerical display of CO_2 concentration, and capnography, which yields a real-time graphic waveform[39]. Ventilation is thus measured as end-tidal CO_2 that approximates $Paco_2$ to within 2–6 mmHg in normal lungs[43]. However, with abnormal cardiopulmonary physiology, the discrepancy is greater. Expired CO_2 is determined[39] by:

(1) Production, dependent on metabolism and varying with temperature and muscle tone;

(2) Transport, dependent on circulation and varying with pulmonary perfusion;

(3) Elimination, dependent on airway and respiratory mechanism integrity.

The premise that, with an intact pulmonary circulation, CO_2 is present in tracheal, but not esophageal gas efflux is thus a reliable method of detecting ETT placement. Presence of CO_2 indicates tracheal intubation, and absence of CO_2 indicates esophageal intubation, circulatory arrest, technical malfunction, circuit disconnection or intraluminal/extraluminal tube obstruction[44,45].

A false-positive result, or an esophageal tube that is determined to be endotracheal, can occur theoretically in the setting of mask ventilation, causing gastric insufflation of CO_2-containing expired gas. Trends noted during studies of esophageal intubation reveal that the volume of gastric CO_2 expired is lower, usually less than 0.7 vol% CO_2[14,27]. The waveform can initially appear normal, but dissipates with successive ventilations, usually three to six[44,46], even under the influence of carbonated beverage consumption[44,47].

A false-negative result, or an endotracheal tube determined to be esophageal, can occur in a low pulmonary blood flow state, specifically cardiac arrest. However, a correlation between end-tidal CO_2 and cardiac output has been demonstrated during cardiopulmonary resuscitation (CPR)[48] with return of circulation[49]. Thus, end-tidal CO_2 monitoring is feasible during cardiac arrest and has even been suggested as a monitor of CPR efficacy[50].

CLINICAL TRIALS

Recent clinical trials that have examined portable devices for confirmation of ETT placement should be scrutinized for two significant points: the prevalence of arrest patients studied and the incidence of false-negative findings that would result in misinterpretation of intratracheal position as equivocal or esophageal in a low-perfusion state. In a controlled trial of 62 patients, Goldberg and co-workers found a colorimetric device (sensitivity 0.03 to 5 vol% CO_2) to be accurate in spontaneously breathing patients with one case (1.6%) of equivocal position that resolved with proper ETT cuff inflation[51].

Studies performed by Ornato and co-workers[52], Bhende and co-workers[53] and Gerard and co-workers[35], which included arrest patients in prehospital and hospital settings, have demonstrated false-negative rates of 23.6% (17 of 72), 18.2% (two of 11) and 31.4% (11 of 35), respectively. Thus, under the most rigorous testing conditions, the colorimetric detector, although effective in patients with spontaneous respirations, has limited sensitivity for detecting intratracheal intubations in the arrest population (Figure 6).

APPARATUS

A miniaturized, infrared, solid-state, end-tidal CO_2 detector was used to confirm emergency ETT placement in a study of 100 intubations in the critically ill by Vukmir and colleagues[54] (Table 1). The indication for airway intervention was considered urgent in 79% and under arrest conditions in 21%. The mean number of intubation attempts was 1.83 (range 1–5) with difficulty of intubation of 6.48 and confirmation of 7.75, on a linear scale from 0 (lowest) to 10 (highest). Determination of ETT position revealed intratracheal intubation in 96% and esophageal intubation in 4%. Placement was confirmed by direct visualization or radiography in all cases. Sensitivity and specificity for ETT localization was 100% ($p < 0.0001$). This hand-held infrared capnometer reliably confirms ETT placement under emergency conditions.

However, in this study, Minicap III had no false-negative results in arrest patients (21 of 100) with low-flow states up to a maximum of 65 min. Respiratory variation did vary with CPR efficacy in several cases. The minimal sensitivity for CO_2 detection was not complicated by false-positive results in the four cases of esophageal intubation. An acknowledged difficulty with all such studies performed in patient care settings is the small number of esophageal intubations available for comparison.

Finally, we have noted a problem with infrared detection of CO_2 in cold weather (less than 0°C), and the device is not currently recommended in the field environment under such conditions[55] (Figure 7).

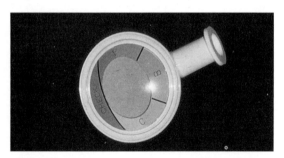

Figure 6 Fenem® end-tidal CO_2 detector (Nellcor)

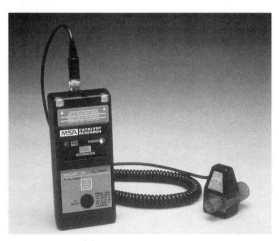

Figure 7 Minicap III® CO_2 detector, (Mine Safety Appliances, Co.)

Table 1 Indication and methods of confirmation of intubations

	% of patients
Indication	
Respiratory distress	31
Airway protection	27
ETT position	18
Cardiac arrest	17
Traumatic arrest	4
ETT replacement	3
Confirmation	
Chest auscultation	98
Epigastric auscultation	92
Chest excursion	87
Chest radiograph	82
Direct visualization	79
Pulse oximetry	67
ETT condensation	36
Arterial blood gas	4

ETT, endotracheal tube

CONCLUSION

Portable qualitative capnometry is a sensitive and specific method of confirming endotracheal tube placement in an emergency in-hospital setting in conjunction with radiographic and clinical information.

References

1. Kastendieck JG. Airway management. In Rosth P, Baker FG, Barken RN, *et al.*, eds. *Airway Management in Emergency Medicine*, 2nd edn. St Louis: CV Mosby, 1988:41–68
2. MacEwen W. Clinical observations on the introduction of tracheal tubes by the mouth instead of performing tracheotomy or laryngotomy. *Br Med J* 1880;2:122–4
3. Jackson C. *Tracheo-bronchoscopy, Esophogoscopy, and Gastroscopy*. St. Louis: St. Louis Laryngoscope Co., 1907
4. Craig J, Wilson ME. A survey of anesthetic misadventures. *Anaesthesia* 1981;36:933–6
5. Utting JE, Gray TC, Shelley JC. Human misadventure in anesthesia. *Can Anaesth Soc J* 1979;26:472–8
6. Solazzi RW, Ward RJ. The spectrum of medical liability cases. *Int Anesthesiol Clin* 1984;22:43
7. Stirt JA. Endotracheal tube misplacement. *Anaesth Intensive Care* 1982;10:274–6
8. Pollard BJ, Juniue FF. Accidental intubation of the esophagus. *Anaesth Intensive Care* 1980;8:183–6
9. Abarhanell NR. Esophageal placement of an endotracheal chest tube by paramedics. *Am J Emerg Med* 1988;6:178–9
10. Frey C, Heulke DF, Gikes PW. Resuscitation and survival in motor vehicle accidents. *J Trauma* 1969;9:292–310
11. Stewart RD, Paris PM, Winter PM. Field endotracheal intubation by paramedic personnel. *Chest* 1984;85:341–5
12. Chaters P, Wilkinson K. Confirmation of tracheal tube placement [Letter]. *Anaesthesia* 1988;43:72
13. Howelle TH, Riethmuller RJ. Signs of endotracheal intubation. *Anaesthesia* 1980;35:984–6
14. Linko K, Palobeim M, Tammisto T. Capnography for detection of accidental esophageal intubation. *Acta Anaesth Scand* 1983;27:199–202
15. Birmingham PK, Cheney FW, Ward RJ. Esophageal intubation: a review of detection techniques. *Anesth Analg* 1986;65:886–91
16. Comroe J, Borelo H. Unreliability of cyanosis in the recognition of arterial anoxemia. *Am J Med Sci* 1947;214:1
17. Triner L. A simple maneuver to verify proper position of an endotracheal tube. *Anesthesiology* 1982;57:548–9
18. Horton WA, Ralston S. Cuff palpation does not differentiate esophageal from tracheal placement of tracheal tubes. *Anaesthesia* 1988;43 (Suppl):803–4
19. Ehrenwerth J, Nagla S, Hirach N, *et al.* Is cuff palpation a useful tool for detecting endotracheal tube position? *Anesthesiology* 1986;65: A137
20. Charters P, Wilkinson K. Tactile orotracheal tube placement test. *Anesthesia* 1987;42:801–7
21. Suerez M, Chediak K, Ershotwsky P, *et al.* Evaluation of a flexible fiberoptic catheter in confirming endotracheal tube placement in the intensive care unit. *Respir Care* 1987;82: 81–4
22. Vinneswaran R, Whitfield JM. The use of a new ultrathin fiberoptic bronchoscope to determine ET tube position in the sick newborn infant. *Chest* 1981;80:174–7
23. Wes MYK. Esophageal detection device. *Anaesthesia* 1988;43:27–9
24. Oleary JJ, Pollard BJ, Ryan MJ. A method of detecting esophageal intubation or confirming tracheal intubation. *Anaesth Intens Care* 1988; 16:299–301
25. McShane AJ, Martin JL. Preoxygenation and pulse oximetry delay detection of esophageal intubation. *J Natl Med Assoc* 1987;79:987–92
26. Yelderman M, New W. Evaluation of pulse oximetry. *Anesthesiology* 1983;39:349–52
27. Guggenberger H, Lens G, Federle R. Early detection of inadvertent esophageal intubation: pulse oximetry vs capnography. *Acta Anesth Scand* 1989;35:112–15
28. Anderson JW, Clark PI, Kafer EN. Use of capnography and transcutaneous oxygen monitoring during outpatient general anesthesia for oral surgery. *J Oral Maxillofac Surg* 1987;45:3–10
29. Stewart RD, Larosee A, Stoy WA. Use of a lighted stylet to confirm correct endotracheal tube placement. *Chest* 1987;86:900–4
30. Jarvis D, Russell DJ. Cuff seal volumes and esophageal intubation. *Anaesth Intens Care* 1988;16:378
31. Bartra AK, Cohn MA. Uneventful prolonged misdiagnosis of esophageal intubation. *Crit Care Med* 1988;11:763–4
32. Goodman LR, Puttman PC. Radiologic evaluation of patients receiving assisted ventilation. *J Am Med Assoc* 1981;245:858–60

33. Blasioger U, Lens G, Kuhn W. Unrecognized endobronchial intubation of emergency patients. *Ann Emerg Med* 1989;18:852–5

34. Rapheal DT, Confrad FU. Ultrasound confirmation of endotracheal tube placement. *J Clin Ultrasound* 1987;15:459–62

35. Gerard J, MacLeod BA, Heller MB, *et al.* Verification of endotracheal intubation using a disposable end tidal CO_2 detector [Abstract]. *Prehosp Dis Med* 1989;4:74

36. Murrin KR. Intubation: procedures and causes of difficult intubation. In Latto IP, Rosen M, eds. *Difficulties in Tracheal Intubation.* Eastborne, Australia: Baillière Tindall/WB Saunders, 1985:75–89

37. Conready PA, Condman LR, Lange F, *et al.* Alteration of endotracheal tube position: flexion and extension of the head. *Crit Care Med* 1976;4:8–12

38. ERCI Technical Assessment Committee. Deaths during general anesthesia. *Tech Anesth* 1985;5:1–10

39. Kalends Z. Capnography during anesthesia and intensive care. *Acta Anesth Belg* 1978;29:3

40. Smith RH, Volpitto PP. Simple methods of determining CO_2 content of alveolar air. *Anesthesiology* 1959;20:702–3

41. Berman IA, Puigiure JJ, Marx CP. The Einstein CO_2 detector. *Anesthesiology* 1984;60:613–14

42. Swerdlow DB. Capnometry and capnography: the anesthesia disaster early warning system. *Semin Anesth* 1986;3:194–205

43. Burton CW. The value of CO_2 monitoring during anesthesia. *Anaesthesia* 1966;21:173–83

44. Garnett AR, Gervin CA, Gervin AS. Capnograph waveforms in esophageal intubation – effect of carbonated beverages. *Ann Emerg Med* 1989;18:387–90

45. Murray IP, Modell JH. Early detection of endotracheal tube accidents by monitoring CO_2 concentration in respiratory gas. *Anesthesiology* 1983;59:344–6

46. Ping STS. Esophageal intubation [Letter]. *Anesth Analg* 1987;66:488

47. Zhinden S, Schupfer G. Detection of esophageal intubation: the cola complication. *Anesth Analg* 1987;66:483

48. Gazmuri RJ, Von Plante M, Weil MH, *et al.* Arterial PCO_2 as an indicator of system perfusion during CPR. *Crit Care Med* 1989;17:237–9

49. Falk JI, Rackow EC, Weil MH. End tidal CO_2 concentration during CPR. *N Engl J Med* 1988;318:607–11

50. Garnett AN, Ornato JF, Gonzaier ER, *et al.* End tidal CO_2 monitoring during cardiopulmonary resuscitation. *J Am Med Assoc* 1987;257:572–5

51. Goldberg JS, Rowie PR, Zehnder JL, *et al.* Colorimetric and tidal carbon dioxide in the prehospital setting [Abstract]. *Ann Emerg Med* 1990;19:452

52. Ornato JP, Zapley TB, Racht EM, *et al.* Multicenter study of end tidal carbon dioxide in the prehospital setting [Abstract]. *Ann Emerg Med* 1990;19:452

53. Bhende MS, Thompson AE, Cook DA. Validity of a disposable end-tidal CO_2 detector in verifying endotracheal tube position in infants and children [Abstract]. *Ann Emerg Med* 1990;19:483

54. Vukmir RB, Heller MB, Stein KL. Confirmation of endotracheal tube placement: a miniaturized infrared qualitative CO_2 detector. *Ann Emerg Med* 1991;20:726–9

55. *Minicap III CO_2 Detector Operation Manual.* Pittsburgh: Mine Safety Appliances Co., 1990:10–11

Laryngotracheal injury from prolonged intubation

4

INTRODUCTION

Endotracheal intubation is a hallmark of critical care intervention in the intensive care unit (ICU) stay. This life-saving intervention can also result in significant adverse sequelae in both acute and chronic settings. Complications of prolonged intubation may be minimized by careful attention to proper endotracheal tube (ETT) design, cuff and fixation issues. Likewise, there is considerable debate over the optimal time of conversion of endotracheal intubation to tracheostomy. Improved ETT design allows maintenance of the airway for approximately 3 weeks or longer, based on the individual patient. Each 3–5 days compared to late (2–3 weeks) tracheostomy is a matter of individual preference, based on weaning strategy and ICU bed utilization.

History

Review of historic records finds Cullen in 1776 describing intubation and artificial ventilation, where 'it is very practicable to introduce directly into the glottis and trachea, a crooked tube, such as a catheter used for a male adult, in concerning the recovery of persons drowned and seemingly dead'[1]. In 1827, de'Etoille described the use of a double-bladed laryngoscope to aid in insertion of such a tube[2]. The modern description of intubation is attributed to MacEwen, who in 1880 suggested the clinical efficacy of the oral endotracheal tube compared to the then current interventions of tracheostomy or laryngotomy[3]. However, widespread use of endotracheal intubation was not performed prior to an extensive treatise on the subject by Chevalier Jackson in 1907[4].

INITIAL COMPLICATIONS

The initial complication rate of airway intervention is addressed by the American Society of Anesthesiologists Closed Claims Project, citing respiratory events in 37% of patients associated with difficult intubation (42%) and a catastrophic outcome – brain injury or death – in 47%, where esophageal intubation has occurred[5]. A Canadian survey of 2000 anesthetists polled over a 7-year period found approximately 600 accidents with esophageal intubation in 30% of cases, which was accompanied by a 46% mortality[6]. The representative incidence of complications is 0.9%, suggested by an analysis of 8000 anesthetic cases[7].

Initial complications in emergency intubation has occurred in 56% of cases, correlated with underlying diagnosis and premorbid condition, but not related to practitioner specialty or level of training[8]. The most frequent complication was dental trauma in patients who were predisposed by previous cosmetic surgery or periodontal disease, involving maxillary incisors, often manifested as fracture of crowns or roots (44%), partial luxation (20%) or avulsion (20%)[9]. Another condition commonly encountered in the early postintubation phase is a sore throat. The incidence of odynophagia ranged from 15% to 60%, correlated in some cases with the presence of a low- or high-pressure cuff model, where intracuff pressure was increased by nitrous oxide diffusion into the cuff[10].

Pharyngoesophageal injury, a more severe complication, is typically found in a hastily performed emergency intubation by inexperienced personnel using a curved ETT or a stylet, with head malposition or cricoid pressure[11]. The syndrome presents with cervical pain, fever, dysphagia, leukocytosis, subcutaneous emphysema or pneumomediastinum[11]. The diagnosis may be made by chest radiograph or bronchoscopy, and therapy consists of tracheostomy and antibiotics[12].

GENERAL COMPLICATIONS

The complications of airway intervention are inevitable, as suggested by a study of 1000 patients extubated after standard operative intervention, demonstrating a 6% rate of severe lesions including hematoma, mucous membrane laceration or subluxation of the arytenoid cartilage[13]. Predisposed patient populations include females and those with smaller stature, diabetes or burns[14,15]. This higher prevalence in females was demonstrated in Realini's study where both functional – dysphonia (48% vs. 18%) – and structural lesions (23% vs. 13%) occurred more commonly in women than men, perhaps due to the ETT and airway size discrepancy[16].

The lesions associated with endotracheal intubation are laryngeal stenosis of the glottic and subglottic region, while tracheostomy can often result in tracheal stenosis in the inferior respiratory tract[17]. Specifically, mucosal ulcerations are found on the posterior-medial vocal cords (94%), not necessarily related to duration of intubation, and most (63%) resolve spontaneously[18]. The incidence approaches 63% for true vocal cord granulomas, 31% for ring-shaped tracheitis at the cuff site, and 10% for tracheal stenosis, with correlations with severe respiratory failure, high cuff pressure and secretion infection related to subsequent complications[19].

Clinical studies have examined particular patient groups. The complication rate in healthy, young patients with traumatic head injury is 61% for intubation and 20% for tracheostomy, and is related to duration of intubation and the pressure of chronic illness – diabetes mellitus, atherosclerotic heart disease and immunosuppression[20]. Pediatric patients demonstrate a higher complication rate with tracheostomy (26%) than orotracheal (10%) or nasotracheal (11%) intubation[21]. Those with closed head injury have a greater complication rate (34%) of long-term airway intervention, mainly vocal cord paralysis, stenosis and tracheomalacia[22]. The complication rate is higher still in those with severe medical illness, equivalent for intubation and tracheostomy in incidence of laryngotracheal injury (95% vs. 91%), but increased tracheal stenosis in those with tracheostomy (19% vs. 65%)[23].

Thus, standard ICU practice has progressed from intubation (44%), using a high-pressure cuff (61%) with monitoring every week (44%), and patients remaining intubated for 7–14 days (50%)[24]. Current standards include oral intubation with a low-pressure cuff with frequent monitoring and an individualized duration of intubation, before conversion to tracheostomy.

The complication rate of airway intervention is related to duration of intubation, with 37% utilized for periods of 1 week or less, while patients intubated for longer than 1 week have a 52% complication rate[25]. Subtle findings such as hoarseness or dysarthria may be found in an even larger proportion (77%) of those receiving tracheostomy[25]. Symptoms expressed by patients are diverse, and include dysphonia (57%), aspiration (25%), dysphagia (23%), odynophagia (21%), dyspnea (21%), stridor (17%) and hoarseness (14%)[26].

Adverse sequelae of endotracheal intubation and tracheostomy may be delineated in incidence (common or rare), and outcome (indolent or catastrophic) (Table 1). Infection is commonly encountered during intubation with most (75%) occurring in the first 2 weeks, more often by basal (40%) than oral (20%) routes[27]. Predisposition is established by the presence of an ETT, where the cuffed more than the uncuffed variety is associated with decreased mucous flow[28]. This decrease in mucociliary clearance is worsened by the administration of anesthetic agents[29]. Nosocomial infection of the tracheobronchial tree often involves Gram-negative bacilli and the incidence is somewhat lessened by adequate humidification[30]. Culture identification of *Klebsiella pneumoniae*, *Staphylococcus aureus*, *Escherichia coli*, *Proteus mirabilis* and *Pseudomonas aeruginosa* helps to differentiate infection from colonization[16].

Table 1 Complications associated with intubation and tracheostomy

	Incidence (%)
Common	
Infection	36
Hemorrhage	36
Aspiration	23
Subcutaneous emphysema	13
Pneumomediastinum	13
Stenosis	11
Air leak	7
Atelectasis	5
Edema	5
Tissue damage	3
Granuloma	3
Pneumothorax	2
Tracheomalacia	1
Rare	
Palate perforation	
Cricoarytenoid subluxation	
Vocal cord paralysis	
Hypopharyngeal perforation	
Tracheal rupture	
Paratracheal abscess	
Tracheal necrosis	
Tracheoinnominate fistulae	
Tracheoesophageal fistulae	

The incidence of nosocomial pneumonia (45%) is highest following emergency intubation, often occurring within 72 h, but without changing mortality or outcome compared to non-emergency intubation[31].

Rarer complications include palate perforation, which has been described secondary to prolonged intubation attempts[32]. Cricoarytenoid subluxation is associated with blind traumatic intubation attempts with a stylet, resulting in fracture of lateral dislocation[33]. Aphonia is the result of decreased vocal cord abduction or cricoarytenoid ankylosis due to long-term endotracheal intubation, which may be treated by vocal cord injection of fludrocortisone or hyaluronidase[34]. Vocal cord paralysis may be caused by intra-arytenoid fibrosis, specifically involving the processus vocalis and posterior commissure, and often treated by endoscopic incision[35]. Pathogenesis suggests involvement of the recurrent laryngeal nerve, which can be interposed in a position between the ETT cuff and thyroid cartilage located 6–10 mm below the true vocal cords[36]. This vocal cord paresis may be unilateral, owing to asymmetric cuff inflation or bilateral, secondary to laryngeal adductor paresis[37,38]. Function may return as the neurapraxia is often temporary.

Catastrophic complications associated with operator inexperience include hypopharyngeal perforation occurring in the pharynx, posterior to the cricopharyngeus muscle or the piriform sinus, requiring early medical and surgical intervention[39]. Tracheal rupture may be found in those predisposed by musculoskeletal conditions such as the rigid spine syndrome[40]. Retropharyngeal abscesses are found after emergency nasotracheal intubation, indicated by rapid onset of fever and odynophagia[41]. Tracheoesophageal space abscess results in bilateral arytenoid fixation and a higher rate of subglottic stenosis[42]. Massive tracheal necrosis is found in those with hypoperfusion, infection or increased cuff pressure resulting in impaired microcirculatory flow; it may be diagnosed by computed tomography, and is usually repaired by end-to-end anastomosis[43,44].

Tracheoarterial erosion syndromes involving the carotid or brachiocephalic trunk often result in rapid patient demise due to asphyxiation more than exsanguination[45]. Patients at risk include those with infection, hypoperfusion, thyromegaly and malnutrition. This complication is caused by anterior tracheal compression and ischemia at the cuff site or tracheostomy tube tip[46]. Diagnosis is suspected in those with more than 10 ml of apparently arterial tracheal bleeding without obvious cause. Acutely, therapy consists of cuff inflation or direct manual compression of the space between the tracheostomy site and manubrium, often followed by orotracheal intubation[46].

Definitive repair involving innominate artery resection or Dacron graft reconstruction is undertaken in the controlled operating-room setting. Tracheoesophageal fistulae can be found acutely in those with traumatic injury, while chronically ventilated patients may demonstrate a more indolent course[47,48].

These conditions require a high index of suspicion to avoid further patient compromise.

However, the most germane issue for routine intensive care practice is an appropriate diagnosis of postintubation or tracheostomy pneumothorax, predominantly unilateral but occasionally bilateral, described in some cases[49].

PATHOLOGY

Complications of prolonged airway support are better understood by analysis of pathological specimens. Most complications may be attributed to the tube or cuff components. The presence of an isolated endotracheal tube segment affixed to canine tracheal mucosa causes erythema at 24 h, progressing to severe mucosal ulceration and loss of airway architecture by 1 week[50]. Similarly, complications occur most commonly below the first tracheal ring, usually stenosis or tracheomalacia at the cuff site[51]. Initial changes are found with slowing of tracheal mucous velocity; the superficial respiratory epithelium may undergo squamous metaplasia[52]. The respiratory epithelium may sustain damage in as little as 4 h of intubation. These early changes consist of flattening, fusion and erosion of respiratory epithelial cells, resulting in compromised ciliary function due to ischemia and mechanical abrasion[53]. The presence of cuff irritation has also resulted in constriction of the smooth muscle of the trachea in 71% of cases, and is blunted by atropine[54].

The tracheal vascular supply localized to the submucosa is oriented in a circumferential direction anteriorly and longitudinally in the posterior portion of the trachea[55]. Capillary perfusion is inversely proportional to extrinsic cuff pressure and is estimated at 22 mmHg (30 cmH$_2$O)[55]. Studies utilizing an endoscopic photographic technique suggest that tracheal blood flow is normal at 25 cmH$_2$O, but the appearance becomes pale at 40 cmH$_2$O, blanched at 50 cmH$_2$O and flow is absent at 60 cmH$_2$O of cuff pressure[55]. Thus, recommendations for extrinsic cuff pressure suggest that flow is initially affected at levels of 30 cmH$_2$O and complete occlusion occurs at 50 cmH$_2$O of cuff pressure[55]. This work has

been validated by hydrogen clearance testing suggesting decreased flow at a transtracheal wall pressure of 3.9 kPa (30 mmHg) and suggests a limit of 2.6 kPa (20 mmHg)[56]. However, there is a biphasic response where normal tracheal blood flow (0.3 ml/min) is increased ten-fold by ETT irritation due to histamine relaxation of arterioles[57]. Again, cuff pressure of 30 mmHg or levels of 20 mmHg localized over cartilage rings may cause significant ischemia[57].

The final endpoint of such ischemia is often tracheal scarring and stenosis. Acquired subglottic stenosis is found in Marshall's canine model experiencing 2 weeks of intubation with unregulated cuff pressure where ulceration was followed by granulomatous change and cicatrix formation[58]. Human studies revealed a 1–8% incidence of such lesions in the subglottic region, beginning with mucosal necrosis and progressing to full thickness erosion, perichondritis and cicatrix proportional to the duration of instrumentation[59].

Clinical outcome studies have demonstrated that most (78%) of the lesions re-epithelialized and healed by 8 weeks, while 9% of patients had a normal laryngeal surface, and 7% were left with granuloma[60]. Retrospective autopsy observations include inflammation of perichondrium of vocal process, cricoid laminae and bacterial invasion beginning at 48 h and progressing to ulceration by 96 h[61]. Comprehensive endoscopic evaluation has suggested inflammation of the true vocal cords (68%), anterior or posterior commissure (29%), false vocal cords (29%), glottis (21%), epiglottic folds (18%) and arytenoid cartilage in 11% of the patients examined[36]. This grading scale described lesions as mild (36%), moderate (24%), severe (22%) and complete subglottic obstruction (15%)[26].

ENDOTRACHEAL TUBE COMPLICATIONS

Complications of endotracheal intubation can be attributed to either the tube or the cuff components. Even the presence of a cuffless tube has resulted in severe laryngeal trauma discovered at autopsy[62]. These effects may be due to ETT characteristics such as size, tip design, composition, position, shape or special characteristics (Figure 1). There is a clear association between endotracheal tube diameter and complications[63,64] (Table 2). This injury is localized to the posterior glottis, where pressures of 200–400 mmHg are exerted by the non-deformable tube, somewhat lessened by a smaller-diameter ETT[65]. This relationship is relative, where the ETT size is compared with the diameter of the trachea[66]. Thus, an 8.0 Fr ETT is acceptable for women, and an 8.5 Fr ETT is more appropriate for the larger trachea in men.

Clinical examination of ETTs of various sizes (6.0, 7.0, 8.0 and 9.0 Fr) suggests that, although wall pressure (0, 18, 8 and 15 mmHg) is decreased by smaller tubes, the seal volume required (23, 58, 54 and 62 mmHg) for effective ventilation may increase as their diameter decreases[67]. Thus, the most effective regimen is an appropriately sized tube relative to the diameter and cuff volume required for an effective seal without overdistension.

The limiting factor in minimizing ETT size and subsequent damage is resistance to flow and imposed work of breathing. There is a somewhat linear relationship between pressure gradient (P) and flow (Q). Modifiers include gas molecule and wall friction, where resistance, R = P/Q. The pressure gradient required to generate gas or liquid flow can be inferred by the Hagen–Poiseuille relationship, where the rapidity of capillary flow is directly proportional to the square of the tube diameter (D) and the pressure (P), and indirectly to the tube length (L), constant (W) and fluid viscosity (V). The suggestion is that laminar flow (expressed by the equation $\Delta p = 8 \times L \times u \times V/\delta R4$) requires less pressure than turbulent flow (expressed by the equation $\Delta p = 8p (L/D)V^2/\delta D4$)[68]. Therefore,

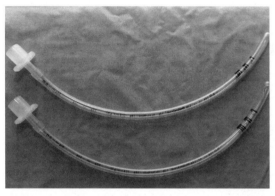

Figure 1 Endotracheal distal tip design. (a) Magill tip (Mallinckrodt, Glen Falls, NY), (b) Murphy tip (Mallinckrodt, Glen Falls, NY)

Table 2 Endotracheal tube sizing. From references 26, 34–50, 173, 183, 184

Endotracheal tube size (French)	Inner diameter (mm)	Approximate outer diameter (mm)	Length (cm)
2.0	2.0	3.0	140
2.5	2.5	3.6	140
3.0	3.0	4.3	160
3.5	3.5	4.9	180
4.0	4.0	5.6	200
4.5	4.5	6.2	220
5.0	5.0	6.9	240
5.5	5.5	7.5	270
6.0	6.0	8.2	280
6.5	6.5	8.9	290
7.0	7.0	9.5	300
7.5	7.5	10.2	310
8.0	8.0	10.8	320
8.5	8.5	11.4	320
9.0	9.0	12.1	320
9.5	9.5	12.8	320
10.0	10.0	13.5	320

the pressure gradient required to generate flow is decreased with an ETT that has a larger diameter, and is shorter and straighter. The position of the ETT in the airway is also significant, with a concentric intratracheal location sufficiently above the carina to prevent obstruction clearly advantageous compared to eccentric positioning[69].

The resistance to flow may be quantified as work of breathing, which is inversely proportional to the tube diameter. Maximum work of breathing quantified as the time–tension index can be associated with the smaller ETT of 6.0–7.0 Fr size, sometimes used for nasal or emergency intubation[70]. The non-elastic work of breathing has been documented to be increased two-fold for the 7.0 Fr tube, and one-fold for the 8.0 Fr tube compared to the 9.0 Fr ETT[71].

The next significant factor is the ETT composition. These devices are tested for safety and designated IT (Implantation Tested) according to the US Pharmacopeia XVII, or Z79-certified by the USA Standards Institute[72]. Tube materials are tested for leeching, adsorption, reactivity, permeation and sterility by tissue implantation and cell culture testing[72]. Major tube components include Teflon (duPont, Garden City, NY), a fluorocarbon offering resiliency along with minimal resistance, and used for strength, simulating the structure of metallic or wire-reinforced tubes[72]. Plastic compounds provide the property of malleability rather than composition, and feature nylon, polyethylene and polyvinyl chloride (PVC) construction[72].

The vast majority of today's ETTs are composed of PVC, offering an optimum mix of strength, but allowing anatomic conformability. Last, elastomers such as silicone rubber offer a soft pliable tube causing little damage, but remaining patent[72]. The first ETT was the red rubber Oxford version, which was sometimes found to collapse upon itself with tube inflation[73]. This complication is less likely with PVC-based tubes, but collapse and obstruction have been described[74].

There are several specialty endotracheal tube types available that deserve discussion. Patients often require a resilient non-collapsible tube

for airway manipulation in difficult otolaryngological surgery. The Oswal–Hunton tube has both a corrugated proximal portion that is malleable, and a distal smooth metallic end that is rigid[75]. Usually, this ETT is converted to the standard variety postoperatively to minimize airway damage. The anode tube is constructed of parallel sheets of latex rubber and wire spiral-bound reinforcement to prevent collapse, and is utilized with the abnormal head position sometimes required for head and neck or neurosurgery. This tube has been associated with obstruction due to cuff inflation or failure to deflate, emphasizing the importance of the preintubation cuff check[76–78]. However, a more commonly encountered difficulty with the anode tube is obstruction due to crimping caused by jaw excursion and occlusion, making ventilation and suction access difficult. This failure requires early tube change to the conventional design, placing the patient at risk in the early postoperative phase (Figure 2).

Flame-resistant ETTs suitable for laser surgery are also associated with higher complication rates than normal tubes due to decreased deformability. Combustion resistance is provided by polytetrafluoroethylene (Teflon) construction and a metallic tape coating, such as copper (BM No. 425 Venture) or silicone–aluminium oxide (Xomed, Jacksonville, FL), in the 'Laser Shielded Tube'[79,80]. These modifications may prevent ignition of the tube

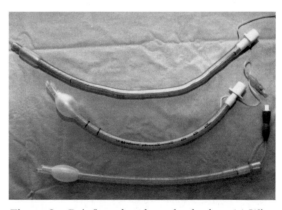

Figure 2 Reinforced endotracheal tubes. (a) Wire reinforced (Rusch, Kernen, Germany), (b) wire reinforced (Mallinckrodt, Glen Falls, NY), (c) laser (Mallinckrodt, Glen Falls, NY)

described as the 'blow-torch' effect, appearing within seconds after laser contact with combustible gas[79,81]. However, these protective modifications can also result in a rigid non-deformable tube that is associated with more frequent nasal and oral complications[80] (Figure 3).

The most promising new development in minimizing the complication rate inherent to the ETT itself is the anatomically shaped tube. This tube design uses an anatomically correct anterior and posterior contour, minimizing posterior deformation forces resulting in laryngeal damage[82]. This relationship was first explored by Lindholm and Carroll, who suggested that deformation forces were minimal with an anatomically shaped tube (30–41 g) compared to PVC (230–296 g) and red rubber (1000 g) tubes, and this difference was accentuated as the ETT size increased[83]. This finding was confirmed clinically when use of the anatomic tube resulted in a decreased incidence of moderate and severe laryngeal injury[84]. Furthermore, the combination of an S-shaped arcuate ETT tube composed of siliconized rubber results in decreased laryngeal loading[85]. However, a recent trial has suggested equivalent arytenoid and tracheal damage, although cricoid damage is still minimized by the Lindholm tube[86] (Figure 4).

Clinical trials of available standard ETTs allow us to draw some conclusions. An evaluation of 500 intubated patients revealed that low cuff pressure, PVC composition and an N_2O diffusion system resulted in fewer complications – voice change or odynophagia with an incidence of 51% and 24%, respectively[87]. Furthermore, the addition of a cuff pressure regulation system resulted in minimal tracheal damage and aspiration compared to the high-volume, low-pressure cuff[88,89]. Thus, the ideal ETT should be soft and thermo-labile, yet resistant to collapse and kinking.

ENDOTRACHEAL TUBE CUFF COMPLICATIONS

Perhaps even more important than the endo-tracheal tube itself, the cuff component has

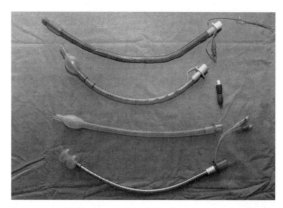

Figure 3 Laser Shielded Tube (Xomed, Jacksonville, FL)

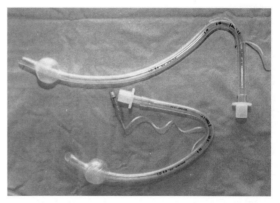

Figure 4 Anatomic design. (a) RAE nasal tube (Mallinckrodt, Glen Falls, NY), (b) RAE oral tube (Mallinckrodt, Glen Falls, NY)

the most significant effect on complications resulting from airway intervention. The static tracheal wall pressure (TWP_s) is the difference between pressure outside (P_o) and pressure inside (P_i) the cuff ($TWP_s = P_o - P_i$). This relationship suggests that when an intracuff pressure of 25 ± 5 cmH$_2$O approximates the tracheal wall capillary perfusion pressure of 30 ± 5 cmH$_2$O, flow may be compromised. The dynamic tracheal wall pressure (TWP_d) is the TWP_s combined with peak airway pressure (PAP), yielding the equation $TWP_d = P_o - P_i + PAP$.

Thus, in the critically ill patient with elevated peak airway pressures transmitted to the cuff, tracheal wall capillary perfusion is often compromised. The importance of peak airway pressure, when monitoring cuff pressure, has been established, since the cuff pressure alone often underestimates the potential damage[90,91]. In addition, the proximal airway pressure does not reflect the distal airway pressure, which is often higher[92]. Clinically, an awake ventilated patient often demonstrates a significant increase in transmitted pressure with oral suctioning (235 ± 69%), endotracheal suctioning (305 ± 29%), coughing (236 ± 80%) and movement (174 ± 65%) over baseline[93].

Cuff damage often manifests as tracheal dilatation with onset between 4 and 8 days, especially with a high-pressure, low-compliance cuff design[94]. Scanning electron microscopy of canine pathological sections documents complete cilia denudation even with a deflated cuff, and mucous damage especially over tracheal rings, even with minimal cuff inflation by 2 h[95]. These changes, which are reversed partially by 2 days of extubation and completely by 1 week, have correlated well with human anatomic specimens[95].

Critically ill patients are at risk for further intubation complications after operative intervention due to nitrous oxide diffusion into the endotracheal cuff, increasing transmitted pressure. This effect occurs when oxygen and nitrous oxide diffuse into the cuff, while nitrogen fails to diffuse out, causing a progressive increase in cuff pressure. Clinical trials have suggested that this effect is minimized in low-pressure, high-volume cuffs and may be prevented by back-filling of the cuff with anesthetic inspired gas[96]. Cuff pressure has been monitored and demonstrated to increase five-fold during operative intervention, suggesting that cuff wall contact is proportional to diffusion[97]. Diffusion is governed by nitrous oxide concentration, cuff wall thickness and surface area of the cuff. Currently available Hi-Lo endotracheal tubes may reach cuff pressures of 100 mmHg within 2 h[98]. The 'rediffusion system' has prevented cuff-resorbed nitrous oxide from diffusing out through an enlarged pilot balloon to maintain cuff pressure increase to less than two-fold by 6 h[98].

Frequent cuff pressure monitoring may be the most effective means of preventing airway complications in the ICU. The simplest method is cuff inflation to leak pressure, where a slight audible air leak is sufficient for ventilation to maintain a cuff pressure of 25 cmH$_2$O[99]. Standard monitoring utilizes a three-way stopcock and a mercury sphygmomanometer to sense cuff pressure, and the pressure-sensitive aneroid (Sims, Keene, NH), which is 99.3% accurate to within 2 mmHg[100]. Direct pressure sensing has been described in research protocols using a Teflon envelope situated between the cuff and tracheal wall, documenting pressures of 0.1–0.3 kPa[101].

The first ETT cuffs utilized were of the low-volume, high-pressure variety. Currently the standard is a high-volume, low-pressure cuff that demonstrates a decreased transmitted lateral wall pressure difference with less mucosal change, inflammation and ulceration[102]. The canine model of Cooper and Grillo suggests that a low-pressure cuff is associated with minimal gross or microscopic lesions, compared to the high-pressure variety, demonstrating circumferential erosion, mucosal ulceration and cartilage destruction[103]. Tracheal wall pressure is due to a complex interaction of ETT size, tracheal diameter, cuff inflation pressure and symmetry, where the large-volume, low-pressure cuff minimizes the deleterious effects of intubation (Figure 5).

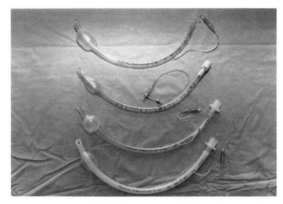

Figure 5 Cuff design. (a) High volume, low pressure (Mallinckrodt, Glen Falls, NY), (b) intermediate volume, pressure (Mallinckrodt, Glen Falls, NY), (c) low volume, high pressure (Mallinckrodt, Glen Falls, NY), (d) Silastic tube composition (Mallinckrodt, Glen Falls, NY)

More moderate approaches suggest that the best cuff may be the intermediate volume variety. There is a suggestion that both large-volume and small-volume cuffs cause equivalent experimental damage[91,104]. The risk of vocal cord cuff herniation with a malpositioned large-volume cuffed tube has been described[105]. Although the enlarged surface area of a high-volume cuff results in less severe damage than the low-volume cuff, there appear to be specific lesions due to redundant excessive cuff folds[89]. The preponderance of evidence suggests that the high-volume cuff should be utilized in most patients, but individual cases may benefit from the intermediate or, in rare circumstances, the low-volume cuff.

The advent of the foam cuff has demonstrated, in canine trials, a decreased incidence of mucosal ischemia, ulceration and cartilage damage[106]. This foam cuff (Bivona, Gary, IN) establishes a tracheal seal from recoil pressure of the material generating $15 \, cmH_2O$ of tracheal wall pressure, even with a negative or zero atmospheric pressure due to the external cuff alone, preventing aspiration without tracheal damage[107]. Trials comparing foam with the high-volume, low-pressure cuff suggest less mucosal damage, demonstrating decreased cuff pressures (0–280 mmHg) and tracheal wall pressure (15–200 mmHg), respectively, for the former[108,109] (Figure 6).

Cuff damage is also minimized by regulation of pressure compared to monitoring alone. McGinnis and Lanz pressure-limiting cuffs allow maximal cuff pressures of only $25 \pm 2 \, cmH_2O$, since excess pressure diffuses out through the pilot balloon[55,110]. Continuous cuff inflation results in an 11% complication rate, which may be minimized by inflating the cuff during inspiration, and deflating during expiration, using a valve–ventilation interphase resulting in minimal complications: tissue damage, aspiration and air leak[111]. The Grieshaber Air System used to maintain intra-ocular pressure has been adapted to regulate cuff pressures in an automatic fashion[112]. However, a canine model demonstrated that continuous inflation and intermittent cuff deflation (5 min every hour) are responsible for similar damage, while inflation to air leak

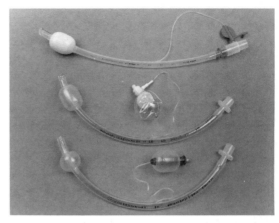

Figure 6 Regulated cuff design. (a) Foam cuff (Bivona, Gary, IN), (b) Brandt cuff (Mallinckrodt, Glen Falls, NY), (c) Lanz cuff (Mallinckrodt, Glen Falls, NY)

is the most effective strategy for minimizing complications[113] (Figure 6).

Another significant cuff complication is aspiration, where fluid pooled above the cuff is followed by a slow downward secretion leak and subsequent pulmonary infection[114]. Interestingly, mechanical ventilation compared to spontaneous ventilation is found to be protective, with the incidence of aspiration decreasing from 100% to 55%[115]. The addition of positive end-expiratory pressure further decreased aspiration from 100% to 15%, as the high-volume cuff may seal with $5–9 \, cmH_2O$[115,116]. Similarly, a cuff system that removes subglottic secretions, the Hi-Lo Evacuation Tube (Mallinckrodt Medical, St Louis, MO) decreases colonization, onset and incidence of pneumonia[117].

Clinical evaluation of cuff design demonstrates that the highest rate of aspiration is found with the low-volume, high-pressure cuff (56%) followed by the intermediate cuff (39%), and the least with the high-volume, low-pressure (20%) design[118]. Although the high-volume, low-pressure cuff minimizes mucosal damage, the aspiration rate may be substantial, owing to redundant cuff folds, ranging up to 100% even with pressures of $50 \, cmH_2O$[119]. Last, the incidence of aspiration is less with endotracheal intubation (0%) compared to tracheostomy (25%)[120].

The basic assumption that cuff pressure underestimates transmitted tracheal wall pressure is correct. This effect is similar for all cuff designs – high-volume, low-volume and foam – and increases 2–17-fold for routine ICU patient interventions[121]. Last, in the critically ill ICU patient, the combined high–low volume, low-pressure cuff reflects increased airway pressure due to decreased lung compliance, which is often significantly greater than intra-cuff pressure[122]. The ideal cuff should be soft and resilient, have high volume with minimal fold redundancy, and occupy a large surface area to provide complete tracheal occlusion.

ENDOTRACHEAL FIXATION

Complications may be minimized by ensuring proper ETT position and fixation. Laryngeal damage is worsened in those who undergo head positioning in extension, excessive suctioning and the agitation found in those who are poorly sedated[83,123]. The extent of intratracheal damage is due to the amount of movement of the endotracheal tube shaft relative to the arytenoids and posterior cricoid, followed by tube tip and the trachea[124,125].

Initial ETT position may be estimated from various anatomic landmarks. The distances from teeth to vocal cords (12–15 cm), vocal cords to carina (10–15 cm) and ETT to carina (male 3.3 cm, female 4.1 cm) are helpful benchmarks[84,126]. Goodman's criteria used clinically suggest a 5 ± 2 cm ETT to carina distance, which has been validated, demonstrating no cases of accidental extubation and a 1% rate of endobronchial intubation[127]. Essential to ICU care is the dynamic description of ETT variability, where head flexion moves the tube 1.9 cm to the carina, extension 1.9 cm away from the carina and lateral rotation, 0.9 cm away from the carina, to suggest the appropriate position to be in the middle third of the trachea[128].

In pediatrics, age + 5 should be the distance from the carina to the distal ETT tip. The depth of insertion from the dental line is 6.5 cm for the premature infant, 9 cm for the term infant, 12 cm for the toddler (2 years) and 17 cm for the adolescent (10 years) or estimated at 2.75 × ETT inner diameter.

ETT fixation should be stable, comfortable and allow emergency access to the patient. The most stable fixation is provided by buccal or oral devices utilized in oral maxillofacial surgery, but often they are uncomfortable to the patient[129,130]. The emergency situation is addressed by ETT fixation using various adhesive tape strategies. The Secure Easy (Inhalation Plastics, Inc., Chicago, IL) fixation device is composed of synthetic wrap and a plastic tube holder. This device has proven superior to adhesive tape in tube displacement measured clinically and radiographically, and by decreasing oro-buccal complications[131]. However, oral cutaneous breakdown may still occur, as with adhesive tape (Figure 7).

NASOTRACHEAL INTUBATION

The issues regarding the nasotracheal intubation route are complex, with a clear dichotomy between those who support and those who reject its use. The procedure has a reasonable overall success rate in 91% with mild complications such as bleeding in 21%; and severe complications such as massive hemorrhage and retropharyngeal perforation in 10%[132]. The study of Danzl and Thomas found a 92% success rate with complications occurring in only 3%, with no long-term laryngeal pathology noted[133] (Figure 8).

The complication rate of nasotracheal intubation is perhaps slightly higher than that in orotracheal intubation. Rare but catastrophic complications have been described. Maxillofacial trauma with dental fracture and obstruction have been found in the trauma patient[134]. Routine nasal intubation may be associated with inferior turbinectomy often with suspected decreased air passage through an obstructed tube[135]. The cribriform plate can be injured with caudad tube orientation or excessive force applied, and this is indicated by cerebrospinal fluid leakage[136]. Traumatic, short-term (1 h) nasal intubation has been associated with both nasal septum

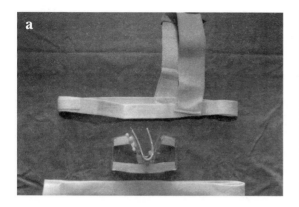

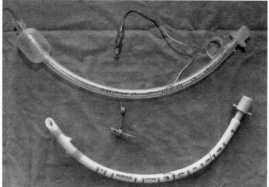

Figure 8 Nasotracheal tube. (a) Endotrol (Mallinckrodt, Glen Falls, NY), (b) silicone (Portex, Keene, NY)

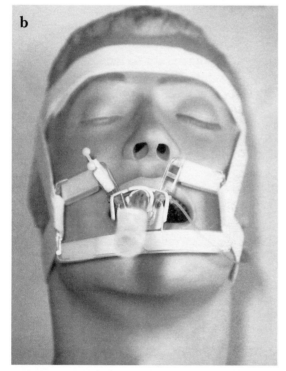

Figure 7 Endotracheal tube fixation. Secure Easy (Inhalation Plastics, Inc., Chicago, IL): (a) device components, (b) device in place

and parapharyngeal abscess[137]. Mediastinal emphysema may develop, usually in conjunction with mucosal ulceration[138].

The most common finding is bleeding, occurring in roughly 45% of patients, usually without adequate nasal mucosa preparation[139]. However, in the ICU, the most important issue is iatrogenic sinusitis. Predisposing factors include decreased nasal mucociliary clearance (65%) detected by a radiopaque disk method

with correlation of difficult or prolonged intubation, often resulting in mechanical trauma to the surface of the epithelium[140]. The incidence of sinusitis is considerably higher with nasal (43%) than oral (2%) tubes[141]. Infection occurs on the ipsilateral side in 42%, and contralateral side in 27% of patients, and requires drainage in 35%, but does not affect mortality adversely[141]. Nasotracheal intubation is most often associated with maxillary or sphenoid (87%) sinusitis, followed by ethmoid (50%) and frontal (12%) disease[142]. The incidence is related to duration of intubation, with 37% affected by 3 days, and 100% involvement by 1 week, with the majority (88%) resolving within 1 week of extubation[142].

The clinical significance of sinusitis needs to be examined in the context of bacteremia and sepsis. The incidence of bacteremia is more common with nasotracheal (29%) than orotracheal intubation (0%), demonstrating aerobic oral flora: *Streptococcus viridans*, *Veillonella* and diphtheroids[143]. True sepsis syndrome occurs in only 7% of those with paranasal sinusitis; it occurs more commonly with emergency (63%) intubation, caused by *Staphylococcus* species compared to elective (37%) cases involving Gram-negative rods[144]. Patients are predisposed by a history of diabetes mellitus or steroid use, while diagnosis is achieved by computed tomography or a Water's View plain radiograph and treated by ETT removal, topical decongestants, antihistamines and antibiotics[145].

There remains ongoing debate concerning the advisability of nasal intubation. The nasal route may be safe for long-term (3–63 days) intubation, and may be associated with half the laryngeal damage of oral intubation[146,147]. However, others have suggested that nasal intubation takes 2.5 times longer than oral intubation and has a significant rate of bleeding (45%) and septicemia (9%) with equivalent comfort, therefore offering no significant advantage[139]. Nasal intubation compared to tracheostomy suggests good experience with the former route that may be maintained for up to 28 days with weekly bronchoscopic surveillance[148]. The incidence of complications in tracheostomy may run as high as 45% with nasal intubation, resulting in decreased incidence and less severity of complications[149]. Therefore, nasal intubation is recommended only on the basis of operator preference and expertise.

ESOPHAGEAL INTUBATION

Although this is infrequently encountered, it is necessary to be aware of the complications associated with placement of esophageal obturator-type ventilation devices. The esophageal obturator device approved in 1973 has undergone clinical use in some three million patients[150,151]. Compared to endotracheal intubation, the esophageal obturator device is easily inserted (6 vs. 20 s) and accurately placed (98% vs. 48%). Placement is a skill easily acquired, providing efficient ventilation and oxygenation[152]. Complications include tracheal intubation and obstruction in 2.9% of patients usually during cardiopulmonary resuscitation followed by aspiration and esophageal or pyriform sinus rupture[151,153]. The device is not commonly employed for hospital-based intubations in light of the risk compared to other alternative methods.

Newer variations on the theme include the Combitube (Sheriden, Argyle, NY) esophageal tracheal tube. This device ventilates independently of esophageal or tracheal position but again, esophageal perforation may be a risk[154]. The pharyngotracheal lumen airway has established efficacy in basic life support care, but suffers from a poor oropharyngeal seal, and esophageal and gastric distension[155] (Figure 9).

DOUBLE-LUMEN ENDOTRACHEAL TUBE

This endotracheal tube was first described by Bjork and Carlens, who developed the double-lumen tube to protect the dependent lung from secretions or bleeding[156]. Robert-Shaw suggested difficulty with placement, and increased resistance with the original Carlens tube compared to his design[157]. Advantages of the double-lumen tube include isolation of the unaffected lung from abscess or hemorrhage, while operating time is reduced[158]. Disadvantages of the double-lumen tube are due to rigidity and include laryngeal and tracheal injury, and left mainstem bronchial rupture indicated by air leak, especially with the Carlens tube[158].

The left-sided tube is positioned with the cuff margin and lumen tip 30 mm apart[159]. The right-sided tube, localized to the mainstem bronchus, has a cuff-to-tip distance of 10 mm, while the right upper-lobe position demonstrates a 15-mm cuff-to-tip distance[159]. Cadaver studies have revealed an estimation of right mainstem distance of 15–19 mm, and left bronchus distance of 44–49 mm for females and

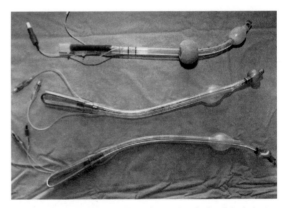

Figure 9 Esophageal and tracheal double-lumen endotracheal tubes. Combitube (Sheriden, Argyle, NY) pharyngo-esophageal airway (double-lumen tubes described in Figure 10)

males, respectively[159]. Fiberoptic confirmation is essential to minimize complications and to suggest a benchmark for left-sided placement of 29 ± 1 cm for each 10 cm of height difference from a 170-cm baseline[160]. The left-sided double-lumen tube is favored because of a decrease in movement (1–8 mm) compared to 16–19 mm for the right-sided tube with a decreased margin of safety[159]. The right-sided endobronchial blocker tube (Sims, Keene, NH) has been found to have equivalent efficacy to the standard double-lumen tube[161]. The tube is utilized postoperatively for independent lung ventilation with separate regulation of ventilatory parameters with differential lung compliance[162] (Figure 10).

The double-lumen tube has been utilized for over 48 000 anesthetic procedures with a 0.4% rate of tracheal rupture, occurring mostly in patients predisposed by tuberculosis or bronchitis, and usually during tube removal[163]. The left-sided tube has been associated with acute right mainstem obstruction, if a decreased carina distance exists[164]. Tracheal rupture has also been reported, even with PVC tubes[165]. Clinical evaluation finds complications such as unsuccessful intubation, dislodgement and malposition manifested as hypoxemia more common in the Carlens (50%) and Robert-Shaw tubes (23%) than the newer PVC tubes[166].

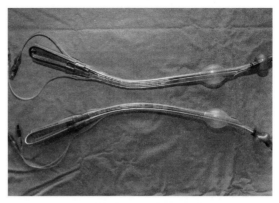

Figure 10 Double-lumen endotracheal tubes. (a) left sided (Mallinckrodt, Glen Falls, NY), (b) right sided (Mallinckrodt, Glen Falls, NY)

ASSESSMENT AND INTERVENTION

The simplest analysis of complications may be by monitoring cuff sizes on the routine chest radiograph[94]. The appearance of an over-distended cuff often precedes tracheal dilatation, subcutaneous emphysema and pneumomediastinum[167]. The most sensitive diagnostic tool is bedside video laryngoscopic assessment, which has been utilized in the intensive care setting demonstrating vocal cord ulceration, subtle motion abnormalities and paresis[168,169]. Historically, xerotomography and tracheography have been supplanted by computed tomography with the capability of diagnosing a wide variety of laryngeal conditions including fracture, dislocation, infection and subcutaneous emphysema[170,171].

The management of postintubation tracheal stenosis includes both medical and surgical approaches. Medical therapy includes steroids: inhaled beclomethasone, intralesional triamcinolone and systemic methylprednisolone associated with peritracheal edema resolution and improved inspiratory and expiratory flow[172,173]. Strategies for progressive dilatation of tracheal stenosis and silicone T-tube stenting have also been described. Surgical therapy has been most successful with resection and end-to-end anastomosis[173].

TIMING OF TRACHEOSTOMY

One of the more controversial issues in intensive care medicine today is the timing of tracheostomy to avoid complications of prolonged intubation. The incidence of complications is strongly correlated with duration of intubation, but prolonged intubation has been tolerated by the nasal route for up to 63 days and the oral route for up to 155 days and even longer in selected patients[146,174,175]. The optimal timing for tracheostomy has been suggested to range from 24 h to 3 weeks based on incidence of complications, with no clear consensus[176–178].

Analysis of tracheostomy timing suggests that patients intubated for less than 3 days in 3%, 3–7 days in 29%, 7–14 days in 50%, 14–21 days in 10%, and more than 21 days in 6%[24].

Thus, the discussion centers upon the 16% of patients intubated for more than 2 weeks[24]. Prospective clinical trials demonstrate a decrease in infectious complications in those with early (5-day) tracheostomy[179]. Mechanical complications are increased in those patients remaining intubated for more than 7 days[180]. The complication rate is minimized for those tracheotomized immediately, with laryngeal damage occurring after 1 week, while pneumonia is more frequent during the second week[181]. However, an early tracheostomy trial (3 days) revealed an eight-fold increase in infection and more frequent tracheal lesions[182].

Each patient's care should be individualized, but it is noted that the complication rate has decreased compared to previous data, due to improved endotracheal tube design. This enables the period of safe intubation to be extended to 2–3 weeks or longer, with the acknowledgement that there is a progressive complication rate as long as the endotracheal tube remains. Therefore, the laryngeal damage of endotracheal intubation must be balanced against early bacterial colonization and perhaps subsequent infection associated with tracheostomy.

The current recommendations suggesting 3 weeks of intubation followed by tracheostomy should be observed and individualized to the patient's premorbid condition, anatomy and clinical outcome.

References

1. Cullen W. A letter to Lord Cathcart, President of the Board of Police in Scotland, concerning the recovery of persons drowned and seemingly dead. London 1776. In *Resuscitation: a Historical Perspective*. Park Ridge, IL: Wood Library Museum, 1976:17
2. d'Etoille LJ. Recherches sur l'asphyxie. *J Phys* 1827. In Huston KG, ed. *Resuscitation: a Historical Perspective*. Park Ridge, IL: Wood Library Museum, 1976:30
3. MacEwen W. Clinical observations on the introduction of tracheal tubes by the mouth instead of performing tracheotomy or laryngotomy. *Br Med J* 1880;2:122–4
4. Jackson C. *Tracheo-bronchoscopy. Esophagoscopy and Gastroscopy*. St. Louis: St. Louis Laryngoscope Co., 1907:1–335
5. Cheney FW, Posner KL, Caplan RA. Adverse respiratory events infrequently leading to malpractice suits. A closed claims analysis. *Anesthesiology* 1991;75:932–99
6. Utting JE, Gray TC, Shelley FC. Human misadventure in anaesthesia. *Can Anaesth Soc J* 1979;26:473–8
7. Craig J, Wilson ME. A survey of anaesthetic misadventures. *Anaesthesia* 1981;36:933–6
8. Taryle DA, Chandler JE, Good JT Jr. Emergency room intubations – complications and survival. *Chest* 1979;75:541–3
9. Bory EN, Goudard V, Magnin C. Tooth injuries during general anesthesia, oral endoscopy and vibro-massage. *Act Odonto-Stomatol* 1991;45:107–20
10. Mandoe H, Nikolajsen L, Lintrup U, *et al*. Sore throat after endotracheal intubation. *Anesth Analg* 1992;74:897–900
11. Tartell PB, Hoover LA, Friduss ME, *et al*. Pharyngoesophageal intubation injuries. *Am J Otolaryngol* 1990;11:256–60
12. Reyes G, Galvis AG, Thompson JW. Esophagotracheal perforation during an emergency intubation. *Am J Emerg Med* 1992; 10:223–5
13. Kambic V, Radsel Z. Intubation lesions of the larynx. *Br J Anaesth* 1978;50:587–90
14. Gaynor EB, Greenberg SB. Untoward sequelae of prolonged intubation. *Laryngoscope* 1985;95: 1461–7
15. Atalic MR, Burke JF. Severe low-pressure cuff tracheal injury in burn patients. *Intensive Care Med* 1981;7:89–92
16. Realini E. Vocal and laryngo-tracheal sequelae of prolonged intubation at the university medical clinic of the Cantonal Hospital at Lausanne. *J Oto-Rhino-Laryngol* 1976;38 (Suppl 1):94–100
17. Hawkins DB. Glottic and subglottic stenosis from endotracheal intubation. *Laryngoscope* 1977;87:339–46
18. Colice GL, Stukel TA, Dain B. Laryngeal complications of prolonged intubation. *Chest* 1989;96:877–84
19. Kastanos N, Miro RE, Perez AM, *et al*. Laryngotracheal injury due to endotracheal intubation: incidence, evolution, and predisposing factors. A prospective long-term study. *Crit Care Med* 1983;11:362–7
20. Lanza DC, Parnes SM, Koltai PJ. Early complications of airway management in head-injury patients. *Laryngoscope* 1990;100:958–61
21. Orlowski JP, Ellis NG, Amin NP, *et al*. Complications of airway intrusion in 100

consecutive cases in a pediatric ICU. *Crit Care Med* 1980;8:324–31

22. Nowak P, Cohn AM, Giudice MA. Airway complications in patients with closed-head injuries. *Am J Otolaryngol* 1987;8:91–6

23. Stauffer JL, Olsen DE, Petty TL. Complications and consequences of endotracheal intubation and tracheotomy. A prospective study of 150 critically ill adult patients. *Am J Med* 1981;70:65–76

24. Pippin LK, Short DH, Bowes JB. Long-term trachea intubation practice in the United Kingdom. *Anaesthesia* 1983;38:791–5

25. Sellery GR, Worth A, Greenway RE. Late complications of prolonged tracheal intubation. *Can Anaesth Soc J* 1978;25:140–3

26. Hsu S, Dreisbach JN, Charlifue SW. Glottic and tracheal stenosis in spinal cord injured patients. *Paraplegia* 1987;25:136–48

27. Boles JM. Upper respiratory tract infections in patients with tracheal intubation. *Rev Practic* 1990;40:2341–3

28. Sackner MA, Hirsch J, Epstein S. Effect of cuffed endotracheal tubes on tracheal mucous velocity. *Chest* 1975;68:774–7

29. Forbes AR, Gamsu G. Lung mucociliary clearance anesthesia with spontaneous and controlled ventilation. *Am Rev Respir Dis* 1979;120:857–62

30. Comer PB, Gibson RL, Weeks DB, *et al.* Airway maintenance in patients with long-term endotracheal intubation. *Crit Care Med* 1976;4:211–14

31. Lowy FD, Carlisle PS, Adams A. The incidence of nosocomial pneumonia following urgent endotracheal intubation. *Infect Control* 1987; 8:245–8

32. Claussen D, Claussen A, Freudenberg J. Perforation of the palate following prolonged orotracheal intubation – a case report. *Anaesthesiol Reanim* 1991;16:333–6

33. Debo RF, Colonna D, Dewerd G, *et al.* Cricoarytenoid subluxation complication of blind intubation with a lighted stylet. *Ear Nose Throat J* 1989;68:517–20

34. Chilla R, Gabriel P. The arthritis of the cricoarytenoid joint, a rare postintubation complication and its novel treatment. *Laryngol Rhinol Otol* 1976;55:389–92

35. Schlondorff G, Elies W. Vocal cord paralysis with stridor caused by interarytenoid fibrosis – a complication of intensive care. *Laryngol Rhinol Otol* 1985;64:403–4

36. Cavo JW Jr. True vocal cord paralysis following intubation. *Laryngoscope* 1985;95:1352–9

37. Gibbin KP, Egginton MJ. Bilateral vocal cord paralysis following endotracheal intubation. *Br J Anaesth* 1981;53:1091–2

38. Hahn FW Jr, Martin JT, Lillie JC. Vocal-cord paralysis with endotracheal intubation. *Arch Otolaryngol* 1970;92:226–9

39. Levin PA. Hypopharyngeal perforation. An untoward complication of endotracheal intubation. *Arch Otolaryngol* 1980;106:578–80

40. Bein T, Lenhart FP, Berger H, *et al.* Rupture of the trachea during difficult intubation. *Anaesthetist* 1991;40:456–7

41. Heath LK, Peirce TH. Retropharyngeal abscess following endotracheal intubation. *Chest* 1977;72:776–7

42. Fee WE Jr, Wilson GG. Tracheoesophageal space abscess. *Laryngoscope* 1979;89:377–84

43. Rubio PA, Farrell EM, Bautista EM. Severe tracheal stenosis after brief endotracheal intubation. *South Med J* 1979;72:1628–9

44. Abbey NC, Green DE, Cicale MJ. Massive tracheal necrosis complicating endotracheal intubation. *Chest* 1989;95:459–60

45. Rinecker H, Schvet T. Arterio-tracheal fistula during long-term intubation of an awake patient. *Anaesthetist* 1979;28:180–1

46. LoCicero J 3d. Tracheo-carotid artery erosion following endotracheal intubation. *J Trauma* 1984;24:907–9

47. Hassenstein J, Schmitt-Koppler A. Tracheo-oesophageal fistula caused by prolonged intubation of a severely injured patient with shock lung syndrome. *Prakt Anaesth Wiederbeleb Intensivther* 1977;12:234–6

48. Payne DK, Anderson W, Romero MD, *et al.* Tracheoesophageal fistula formation in intubated patients: risk factors and treatment with high-frequency jet ventilation. *Chest* 1990;98:161–4

49. Biswas C, Jana N, Maitra S. Bilateral pneumothorax following tracheal intubation. *Br J Anaesth* 1989;62:338–9

50. Bishop MJ, Hibbard AJ, Fink BR. Laryngeal injury in a dog model of prolonged endotracheal intubation. *Anesthesiology* 1985;62:770–3

51. Windsor HM, Shanahan MX, Cherian K. Tracheal injury following prolonged intubation. *Aust NZ J Surg* 1976;46:18–25

52. Belson TP. Cuff induced tracheal injury in dogs following prolonged intubation. *Laryngoscope* 1983;93:549–55

53. Schmidt WA, Schaap RN, Mortensen JD. Immediate mucosal effects of short-term, soft-cuff, endotracheal intubation. A light and scanning electron microscopic study. *Arch Pathol Lab Med* 1979;103:516–21

54. Nishino T, Sugimori K, Hiragi K, *et al.* Effects of tracheal irritation and hypercapnia on tracheal smooth muscle in humans. *J Appl Physiol* 1990;69:419–23

55. Seegobin RD, van Hasselt GL. Endotracheal cuff pressure and tracheal mucosal blood flow: endoscopic study of effects of four large volume cuffs. *Br Med J* 1984;288:965–8

56. Joh S, Matsuura H, Kotani Y, *et al.* Change in tracheal blood flow during endotracheal

intubation. *Acta Anaesthesiol Scand* 1987;31: 300–4

57. Nordin U, Lindholm CE, Wolgast M. Blood flow in the rabbit tracheal mucosa under normal conditions and under the influence of tracheal intubation. *Acta Anaesthesiol Scand* 1977;21:81–94

58. Marshak G, Doyle WJ, Bluestone CD. Canine model of subglottic stenosis secondary to prolonged endotracheal intubation. *Laryngoscope* 1982;92:805–9

59. Gould SJ, Howard S. The histopathology of the larynx in the neonate following endotracheal intubation. *J Pathol* 1985;146:301–11

60. Colice GL. Resolution of laryngeal injury following translaryngeal intubation. *Am Rev Respir Dis* 1992;145:361–4

61. Donnelly WH. Histopathology of endotracheal intubation: an autopsy study of 99 cases. *Arch Pathol* 1969;88:511–20

62. Trim CM. Complications associated with the use of the cuffless endotracheal tube in the horse. *J Am Vet Med Assoc* 1984;185:541–2

63. Strong RM, Passy V. Endotracheal intubation. Complications in neonates. *Arch Otolaryngol* 1977;103:329–35

64. Santos PM, Afrassiabi A, Weymuller EA Jr. Prospective studies evaluating the standard endotracheal tube and a prototype endotracheal tube. *Ann Otol Rhinol Laryngol* 1989; 98:935–40

65. Weymuller EA, Bishop MJ, Hibbard AW, *et al.* Quantification of intralaryngeal pressure exerted by endotracheal tubes. *Ann Otol Rhinol Laryngol* 1983;92:444–7

66. Black AMS, Seegobin RD. Pressures on endotracheal tube cuffs. *Anaesthesia* 1981;36:498–511

67. Lee TS. Routine monitoring of intracuff pressure. *Chest* 1992;102:1309–10

68. Habib MP. Physiologic implications of artificial airways. *Chest* 1989;96:180–4

69. Menon AS, Weber ME, Chang HK. Velocity profiles in central airways with endotracheal intubation: a model study. *J Appl Physiol* 1986; 60:876–84

70. Shapiro M, Wilson RK, Casar G, *et al.* Work of breathing through different sized endotracheal tubes. *Crit Care Med* 1986;14: 1028–31

71. Plost GN, Campbell SC, Vagedes RT, *et al.* The nonelastic work of breathing by normal human beings using different size endotracheal tubes. *J Intensive Care Med* 1990;5:23–5

72. Stetson JB, Guess WL. Causes of damage to tissues by polymers and elastomers used in the fabrication of tracheal devices. *Anesthesiology* 1970;33:635–52

73. Hoffman S, Freedman M. Delayed lumen obstruction in endotracheal tubes. *Br J Anaesth* 1976;48:1025–8

74. Roland P, Stovner J. Brain damage following collapse of a polyvinyl tube: elasticity and permeability of the cuff. *Acta Anaesthesiol Scand* 1975;19:303–9

75. Hunton J, Oswal VH. Metal tube anaesthesia for ear, nose and throat carbon dioxide laser surgery. *Anaesthesia* 1985;40:1210–12

76. Niederman MS, Ferranti RD, Zeigler A, *et al.* Respiratory infection complicating long-term tracheostomy. *Chest* 1984;85:39–44

77. Malone BT. A complication of Rusch armored endotracheal tubes. *Anesth Analg* 1975;54:756

78. Reddy KD, Naraghi M, Adriani J. Complications from unrecognized defects in endotracheal tubes. *South Med J* 1978;71:783–5

79. Sosis MB. What is the safest endotracheal tube for Nd-YAG laser surgery? A comparative study. *Anesth Analg* 1989;69:802–4

80. Vitkun SA, Sidhu US. Intranasal trauma caused by a sharp-edged laser-resistant (silicone) endotracheal tube. *Anesthesiology* 1985;62:834–5

81. Green JM, Gonzalez RM, Sonbolian N, *et al.* The resistance to carbon dioxide laser ignition of a new endotracheal tube, Xomed Laser-Shield II. *J Clin Anesth* 1992;4:89–92

82. Alexopoulos C, Larsson SG, Lindholm CE. Anatomical shape of the airway. *Acta Anaesthesiol Scand* 1983;27:185–92

83. Lindholm CE, Carroll RG. Evaluation of tube deformation pressure *in vitro*. *Crit Care Med* 1975;3:196–9

84. Lindholm CE. Experience with a new orotracheal tube. *Acta Otolaryngol* 1973;75: 389–90

85. Steen JA, Lindholm CE, Brdlik CG. Tracheal tube forces on the posterior larynx: index of laryngeal loading. *Crit Care Med* 1982;10:186–9

86. Eckerbom B, Lindholm CE, Alexopoulos C. Airway lesions caused by prolonged intubation with standard and with anatomically shaped tracheal tubes. A post-mortem study. *Acta Anaesthesiol Scand* 1986;30:366–73

87. Lipp M, Brandt L, Daublander M. Frequency and severity of throat complaints following general anesthesia with the insertion of various endotracheal tubes. *Anaesthetist* 1988;37:758–66

88. Petring OU, Adelhoj B, Jensen BN, *et al.* Prevention of silent aspiration due to leaks around cuffs of endotracheal tubes. *Anesth Analg* 1986;65:777–80

89. Loeser EA, Hodges M, Gliedman J, *et al.* Tracheal pathology following short-term intubation with low- and high-pressure endotracheal tube cuffs. *Anesth Analg* 1978;57: 577–9

90. Black AM, Seegobin RD. Pressures on endotracheal tube cuffs. *Anaesthesia* 1981;36:498–511

91. Homi J, Notcutt W, Jones JJ, *et al.* A method for comparing endotracheal cuffs. A controlled

study of tracheal trauma in dogs. *Br J Anaesth* 1978;50:435–44

92. Badenhorst CH. Changes in tracheal cuff pressure during respiratory support. *Crit Care Med* 1987;15:300–2

93. Ao EL. Continuous dynamic record of intracuff pressure in endotracheal intubated patients. *Kao-Hsiung I Hsueh o Hsueh Tsa Chih* 1991;7:1–6

94. Honig EG, Francis PB. Persistent tracheal dilatation: onset after brief mechanical ventilation with a 'soft-cuff' endotracheal tube. South Med J 1979;72:487–90

95. Klainer AS, Turndorf H, Wu W, *et al*. Surface alterations due to endotracheal intubation. *Am J Med* 1975;58:674–83

96. Stanley TH, Liu WS. Tracheostomy and endotracheal tube cuff volume and pressure changes during thoracic operations. *Ann Thorac Surg* 1975;20:144–51

97. Brandt L, Pokar H, Ren D, *et al*. Cuff pressure changes due to diffusion of nitrous oxide. A contribution to the question of the *in vivo*-diffusion area of the cuff. *Anaesthetist* 1982;31:345–8

98. Brandt L, Pokar H. The rediffusion system. Limitation of nitrous oxide increases the cuff pressure of endotracheal tubes. *Anaesthetist* 1983;32:459–64

99. Spear RM, Sauder RA, Nichols DG. Endotracheal tube rupture, accidental extubation, and tracheal avulsion: three airway catastrophes associated with significant decrease in leak pressure. *Crit Care Med* 1989;17:701–3

100. Bouvier JR. Measuring tracheal tube cuff pressures – tool and technique. *Heart Lung* 1981;10:686–90

101. Lomholt N. A device for measuring the lateral wall cuff pressure of endotracheal tubes. *Acta Anaesthesiol Scand* 1992;36:775–8

102. Honeybourne D, Costello JC, Barham C. Tracheal damage after endotracheal intubation: comparison of two types of endotracheal tubes. *Thorax* 1982;37:500–2

103. Cooper JD, Grillo HC. Experimental production and prevention of injury due to cuffed tracheal tubes. *Surg Gynecol Obstet* 1969;1235–41

104. Homi J, Notcutt W, Jones J, *et al*. A method for comparing endotracheal cuffs. *Br J Anaesth* 1978;50:435–44

105. Treffers R, de Lange JJ. An unusual case of cuff herniation. *Acta Anaesthesiol Belg* 1989;40:87–90

106. Weymuller EA Jr. Laryngeal injury from prolonged endotracheal intubation. *Laryngoscope* 1988;98(Suppl 45):1–15

107. Power KJ. Foam cuffed tracheal tubes: clinical and laboratory assessment. *Br J Anaesth* 1990;65:433–7

108. Lederman DS, Klein EF, Drury WD, *et al*. A comparison of foam and air-filled endotracheal-tube cuffs. *Anesth Analg* 1974;53:521–6

109. Kamen JM, Wilkinson CJ. A new low-pressure cuff for endotracheal tubes. *Anesthesiology* 1971;34:482–5

110. McGinnis GE, Shively JG, Patterson RL, *et al*. An engineering analysis of intratracheal tube cuffs. *Anesth Analg* 1971;50:557–64

111. Lev A, Barzilay E. Synchronized intermittent mandatory insufflation of the endotracheal tube cuff. *Intensive Care Med* 1983;9:291–3

112. Vitkun SA, Lagasse RS, Kyle T, *et al*. Application of the Grieshaber air system to maintain endotracheal tube. *J Clin Anesth* 1990;2:45–7

113. Hanson B. The effectiveness of hourly cuff deflation in minimizing tracheal damage. *Heart Lung* 1976;5:734–41

114. Whiffler K, Andrew WK, Thomas RG. The hazardous cuffed endotracheal tube – aspiration and extubation. *South Afr Med J* 1982;61:240–1

115. Janson BA, Poulton TJ. Does PEEP reduce the incidence of aspiration around endotracheal tubes? *Can Anaesth Soc J* 1986;33:157–61

116. Nordin U, Lyttkens L. New parachute cuff and positive end-expiratory pressure to minimize tracheal injury and prevent aspiration. *Arch Otol Rhinol Laryngol* 1979;222:119–25

117. Mahul P, Auboyer C, Jospe R, *et al*. Prevention of nosocomial pneumonia in intubated patients: respective role of mechanical subglottic secretions drainage and stress ulcer prophylaxis. *Intensive Care Med* 1992;18:20–5

118. Spray SB, Zuidema GD, Cameron JL. Aspiration pneumonia; incidence of aspiration with endotracheal tubes. *Am J Surg* 1976;131:701–3

119. Seegobin RD, van Hasselt GL. Aspiration beyond endotracheal cuffs. *Can Anaesth Soc J* 1986;33:273–9

120. Lien TC, Wang JH. Incidence of pulmonary aspiration with different kinds of artificial airways. *Chung Hua i Hsueh Tsa Chih* 1992;49:348–53

121. MacKenzie CF, Klose S, Browne DR. A study of inflatable cuffs on endotracheal tubes. Pressures exerted on the trachea. *Br J Anaesth* 1976;48:105–9

122. Guyton D, Banner MJ, Kirby RR. High-volume, low-pressure cuff: are they always low pressure? *Chest* 1991;100:1076–81

123. Schultz-Coulon HJ. Prolonged endotracheal intubation or tracheostomy in children. *Halls Nasen Ohrenheilkund* 1976;24:283–8

124. Whited RE. A study of endotracheal tube injury to the subglottis. *Laryngoscope* 1985;95:1216–19

125. Neumann OG. Parameters of trauma at posterior subglottic region by long term translaryngeal intubation. *Prakt Anaesth Wiederbeleb Intensivther* 1975;10:135–8

126. Stone DJ, Bogdonoff DL. Airway considerations in the management of patients requiring long-term endotracheal intubation. *Anesth Analg* 1992;74:276–87

127. Owen RL, Cheney FW. Endobronchial intubation: a preventable complication. *Anesthesiology* 1987;67:255–7

128. Conrardy PA, Goodman LR, Lainge F, *et al.* Alteration of endotracheal tube position. *Crit Care Med* 1976;4:8–12

129. Richard P, Perier JF, Marsol P, *et al.* Intrabuccal fixation technique for oral intubation catheters. *Rev Stomatol Chir Maxillo-Faciale* 1986;87:402–4

130. Hansen RH, Remensnyder JP. External fixation of endotracheal tubes while skin grafting severe burns of the face. *Plast Reconstruct Surg* 1978;62:628–9

131. Tasota FJ, Hoffman LA, Zullo TG. Evaluation of two methods used to stabilize oral endotracheal tubes. *Heart Lung* 1987;16:140–6

132. Tintinalli JE, Claffey J. Complications of nasotracheal intubation. *Ann Emerg Med* 1981;10:142–4

133. Danzl DF, Thomas DM. Nasotracheal intubations in the emergency department. *Crit Care Med* 1980;8:677–82

134. Kenney JN, Laskin DM. Nasotracheal tube obstruction from a central incisor. Report of a case. *Oral Surg Oral Med Oral Pathol* 1989;67:266–7

135. Wilkinson JA, Mathis RD, Dire DJ. Turbinate destruction – a rare complication of nasotracheal intubation. *J Emerg Med* 1986;4:209–12

136. Young RF. Cerebrospinal fluid rhinorrhea following nasogastric intubation. *J Trauma* 1979;19:789–91

137. Hariri MA, Duncan PW. Infective complications of brief nasotracheal intubation. *J Laryngol Otol* 1989;103:1217–18

138. Nakajima M, Lee YE, Nakazawa T, *et al.* Pneumothorax, subcutaneous emphysema and mediastinal emphysema in transnasally intubated patients. *Nippon Geka Hokan-Archiv Jpn Chir* 1989;58:522–6

139. Depoix JP, Malbezin S, Videcoq M, *et al.* Oral intubation v. nasal intubation in adult cardiac surgery. *Br J Anaesth* 1987;59:167–9

140. Elwany S, Mekhamer A. Effect of nasotracheal intubation on nasal mucociliary clearance. *Br J Anaesth* 1987;59:755–9

141. Saylord F, Gaussorgues P, Marti-Flich J, *et al.* Nosocomial maxillary sinusitis during mechanical ventilation: a prospective comparison of orotracheal versus the nasotracheal route for intubation. *Intensive Care Med* 1990;16:390–3

142. Fassoulaki A, Pamouktsoglou P. Prolonged nasotracheal intubation and its association with inflammation of paranasal sinuses. *Anesth Analg* 1989;69:50–2

143. Cannon LA, Gardner W, Treen L, *et al.* The incidence of bacteremia associated with emergent intubation: relevance to prophylaxis against bacterial endocarditis. *Ohio Med* 1990;86:596–9

144. Deutschman CS, Wilton P, Sinow J, *et al.* Paranasal sinusitis associated with nasotracheal intubation: a frequently unrecognized and treatable source of sepsis. *Crit Care Med* 1986;14:111–14

145. Kronberg FG, Goodwin WJ Jr. Sinusitis in intensive care unit patients. *Laryngoscope* 1985;95:936–8

146. Glumcher FS, Treshchinskii AI, Kravchenko EP, *et al.* Clinical use of long-term nasotracheal intubation. *Anesteziol Reanim* 1989;1:42–4

147. Dubick MN, Wright BD. Comparison of laryngeal pathology following long-term oral and nasal endotracheal intubations. *Anesth Analg* 1978;57:663–8

148. Heovener B, Henneberg U. Limitation of prolonged nasotracheal intubation. *Anaesthetist* 1975;24:529–33

149. Miller JD, Kapp JP. Complications of tracheostomies in neurosurgical patients. *Surg Neurol* 1984;22:186–8

150. Michael TA. The role of the esophageal obturator airway in cardiopulmonary resuscitation. *Circulation* 1986;74:134–7

151. Gertler JP, Cameron DE, Shea K, *et al.* The esophageal obturator airway: obturator or obtundator? *J Trauma* 1985;25:424–6

152. Don Michael TA. Esophageal obturator airway. *Med Instrum* 1977;11:331–3

153. Johnson KR Jr, Genovesi MG, Lassar KH. Esophageal obturator airway; use and complications. *J Am Coll Emerg Physicians* 1976;5:36–9

154. Bigenzahn W, Pesau B, Frass M. Emergency ventilation using the Combitube in cases of difficult intubation. *Eur Arch Otol Rhinol Laryngol* 1991;248:129–31

155. McMahan S, Ornato JP, Racht EM, *et al.* Multi-agency, prehospital evaluation of the pharyngeo-tracheal lumen (PTL) airway. *Prehosp Disast Med* 1992;7:13–18

156. Bjork VO, Carlens E. The prevention of spread during pulmonary resection by the use of a double-lumen catheter. *J Thorac Surg* 1950;20:151–7

157. Robert-Shaw FL. Low resistance double lumen endobronchial tubes. *Br J Anaesth* 1962;34:576

158. Joos D, Zeiler D, Muhrer K, *et al*. Bronchial rupture. Diagnosis and therapy of a rare complication of the use of double-lumen tubes. *Anaesthetist* 1991;40:291–3

159. Benumof JL, Partridge BL, Salvatierra C, *et al*. Margin of safety in positioning modern double-lumen endotracheal tubes. *Anesthesiology* 1987;67:729–38

160. Brodsky JB, Benumof JL, Ehrenwerth J, *et al*. Depth of placement of left double-lumen endobronchial tubes. *Anesth Analg* 1991;73: 570–2

161. Trazzi R, Nazari S. Clinical experience with a new right-sided endobronchial tube in left main bronchus surgery. *J Cardiothorac Anesth* 1989;3:461–4

162. Gallagher TJ, Banner MJ, Smith RA. A simplified method of independent lung ventilation. *Crit Care Med* 1980;8:396–9

163. Lobo Sanchez M, Reinaldo Lapuerta JA, Tamame Tamame C, *et al*. Tracheobronchial lesions due to anesthetic procedures. Report of 2 cases. *Rev Esp Anestesiol Reanim* 1991; 38:51–4

164. Homann B. Acute right bronchial blockade following intubation with a left-swing Robert Shaw tube. *Anaesthetist* 1985;34:91–2

165. Burton NA, Fall SM, Lyons T, *et al*. Rupture of the left main-stem bronchus with a polyvinylchloride double-lumen tube. *Chest* 1983;83:928–9

166. Burton NA, Watson DC, Brodsky JB, *et al*. Advantages of a new polyvinyl chloride double-lumen tube in thoracic surgery. *Ann Thorac Surg* 1983;36:78–84

167. Rollins RJ, Tocino I. Early radiographic signs of tracheal rupture. *Am J Roentgenol* 1987; 148:695–8

168. Alessi DM, Hanson DG, Berci G. Bedside video laryngoscopic assessment of intubation trauma. *Ann Otol Rhinol Laryngol* 1989;98: 586–90

169. Wey W. Injury to the larynx and trachea following artificial respiration. *Schweiz Med Wochenschr J Suisse Med* 1985;115:194–6

170. Dudley JP, Mancuso AA, Fonkalsrud EW. *Arytenoid Otolaryngol* 1984;110:483–4

171. Vukanovic S, Sidani AH, Ducommun JC, *et al*. Tracheal and subglottic lesions following long-standing intubation. A radiological and clinical study. *Diagn Imag* 1982;51:224–33

172. Braidy J, Breton G, Clement L. Effect of corticosteroids on post-intubation tracheal stenosis. *Thorax* 1989;44:753–5

173. Maniglia AJ. Conservative surgical management of tracheal stenosis. *Otolaryngology* 1978; 86:380–93

174. Rashkin MC, Davis T. Acute complications of endotracheal intubation. Relationship to reintubation, route, urgency, and duration. *Chest* 1986;89:165–7

175. Via-Reque E, Rattenborg CC. Prolonged oro- or nasotracheal intubation. *Crit Care Med* 1981;9:637–9

176. Berlauk JF. Prolonged endotracheal intubation vs. tracheostomy. *Crit Care Med* 1986; 14:742–5

177. Marek K, Golebiowska D, Klopotowski J, *et al*. Complications of endotracheal intubation in patients treated for acute poisoning. *Anaesth Resuscitation Intensive Ther* 1975;3:173–9

178. Marsh HM, Gillespie DJ, Baumgartner AE. Timing of tracheostomy in the critically ill patient. *Chest* 1989;96:190–3

179. Dayal VS, El Masri W. Tracheostomy in intensive care setting. *Laryngoscope* 1986;96: 58–60

180. Whited RE. A prospective study of laryngotracheal sequelae in long-term intubation. *Laryngoscope* 1984;94:367–77

181. Fuchs HH, Flugel KA, Druschky KF. Tracheotomy or intubation? Problems with long-term intensive care patients. *Dtsch Med Wochenschr* 1981;106:1022–5

182. El-Naggar M, Sadagopan S, Levine H, *et al*. Factors influencing choice between tracheostomy and prolonged translaryngeal intubation in acute respiratory failure: a prospective study. *Anesth Analg* 1976;55: 195–201

183. Rivera R, Tibballs J. Complications of endotracheal intubation and mechanical ventilation in infants and children. *Crit Care Med* 1992; 20:193–9

184. Aass AS. Complications to tracheostomy and long-term intubation: a follow-up study. *Acta Anaesthesiol Scand* 1975;19:127–33

Surgical airway procedures 5

INTRODUCTION

The absolute indications for intubation include airway obstruction, apnea and respiratory distress. Urgent indications include mental status alteration, trauma, thoracic, mechanical disadvantage or to aid in secretion clearance, oromaxillofacial trauma and diagnostic procedures (Table 1). The need for surgical airway is evaluated in the light of difficulties associated with emergency intubation in the presence of laryngotracheal trauma.

Emergency intubation, often accompanied by muscle relaxation with vecuronium (59%), is accomplished by the oral route in 57%, the nasal route in 40% and cricothyroidotomy in 3% of patients[1]. This procedure is safe, even with cervical fracture found in 7% of trauma patients evaluated by Redan and colleagues, without demonstrating new neurological deficits, but is occasionally accompanied by aspiration (1%)[1]. The procedure is efficacious (97%) with failures occurring in those patients with facial fracture[1]. Patients may also undergo intubation facilitated by succinylcholine, with success on the first attempt in 86%, and in 7% on the second or third, but, in Murphy-Macabobby's evaluation, 3.5% of patients may require surgical airway[2].

The use of neuromuscular blockade has been recommended to assist in difficult intubation, but it is associated with a 6% failure rate, requiring surgical intervention[3]. Muscle relaxation may optimize conditions for oral

Table 1 Airway intervention: intubation, cricothyroidotomy, transtracheal and tracheostomy[187–189]

Intubation	Cricothyroidotomy	Transtracheal intervention	Tracheostomy
Indications			
Airway obstruction	Failed intubation	Failed intubation	Failed cricothyroidotomy
Respiratory distress	Upper airway obstruction	Cervical fracture	Upper airway obstruction
Respiratory mechanics	Secretion clearance	Partial airway obstruction	Long-term mechanical
Hemorrhage	Long-term ventilation	Pharyngeal foreign body	ventilation
Secretion clearance	Recent sternotomy		Difficult weaning
Mental status alteration	Cervical fracture		Decrease ETT injury
Pulmonary contusion	Facial trauma (severe)		Speech capability
Facial trauma			Oral intake
(moderate)			Psychosocial benefit
Diagnostic procedures			Oromaxillofacial trauma
Penetrating neck			Pharyngeal glottic edema
trauma			Nasal oral hemorrhage
Cardiac instability			Neurological damage
Contraindications			
Anatomic difficulty	Laryngeal infection	Complete airway	Recent sternotomy
Coagulopathy (nasal)	Laryngeal trauma	obstruction	'Emergency airway access'
Facial fracture (nasal)	Intubation (3 days)	Pediatric (relative)	
	Pediatric (relative)	Laryngeal trauma	
	Coagulopathy		

ETT, endotracheal tube

intubation (92% vs. 61%) or nasal intubation (60%) accompanied by a defined failure rate of 6% requiring cricothyroidotomy[4]. Lastly, blind nasotracheal intubation has been suggested to be effective (63–72%) for tenuous spontaneously breathing patients, but often requires multiple attempts and is associated with a 13% complication rate[5]. The surgical airway is often considered in emergency cases of suspected cervical spine fracture or severe anatomic deformity associated with oromaxillo-facial or laryngeal disruption.

Perioperative intubation of those with known cervical fracture under optimum conditions demonstrates new neurological deficits in 1.3–2.4% of patients with no differences based on technique (awake or induction), or route (oral or nasal)[6,7]. Most (61%) cervical fractures encountered today occur in motor vehicle accidents. These occurred at the C_1 (7.1%), C_2 (12.1%), C_3 (5.7%), C_4 (15.0%), C_5 (29.2%), C_6 (27.0%) and C_7 (3.5%) vertebrae[8]. These patients were intubated in the operating room by the nasal (71%) and oral (22%) routes, in the emergency department (6%), or in the prehospital realm, all successfully, without new neurological deficit[8].

The incidence of cervical fracture in blunt trauma is 6%. In mostly unstable conditions, patients underwent oral intubation in 49% and nasal intubation in 47% of cases[9]. The need for cricothyroidotomy has been encountered in 4% of patients and new postintubation neurological deficits were documented in 1.9% who underwent nasal intubation[9]. Prevention of further spinal cord trauma may be enhanced by axial in-line stabilization. Distraction of cervical segments up to 7.75 mm as well as posterior subluxation have been noted[10]. Complications may be minimized by expertise, with the experienced operator using decreased force (22 vs. 28 N) and duration (19 vs. 40 s) of the attempt[11]. The blade design bears no influence on cervical spine movement; however, in-line stabilization decreases unnecessary cervical displacement[12]. Thus, emergency intubation may be facilitated by an experi-enced operator, using nasal or oral intubation with muscle relaxants accompanied by in-line stabilization.

The presence of severe laryngotracheal trauma often requires the establishment of surgical airway. Laryngotracheal trauma occurs more commonly with penetrating injury (65%) and is associated with airway compromise (43%) and increased mortality (12%)[13]. The injury may be localized to the larynx, presenting with vocal cord dysfunction manifested as dysphonia; to the cervical trachea (14%), presenting with subcutaneous emphysema; or to the thoracic trachea (54%), diagnosed by pneumomediastinum and hemoptysis[14,15]. Laryngeal injury is a relative contraindication to cricothyroidotomy, so oral–nasal (23%) intubation or tracheostomy (18%) should be chosen to secure an airway[14]. Airway control should be achieved by the most expeditious means possible, usually crico-thyroidotomy, but 'emergency' tracheostomy, a procedure often time consuming even in expert hands, may be performed in extreme circumstances[13–15].

A surgical airway is required in 3.5–6.0% of emergency airway control events, especially with failed intubation, oromaxillofacial trauma, cervical fracture and selected cases of laryngo-tracheal trauma. Cricothyroidotomy is the procedure of choice in the emergency setting with an increased success rate compared to tracheostomy and improved patient neuro-logical outcome based on decreased time required for the procedure[16]. Tracheostomy, if required acutely, is associated with an adverse effect on mortality, due to late intervention[17].

ANATOMY

The surgical airway requires knowledge of anatomic detail (Figure 1). The most superior identifiable external landmark is the hyoid bone connected by the thyrohyoid membrane to the thyroid cartilage, the most readily located structure. The thyroid cartilage is superior to the cricothyroid cartilage, connected by the cricothyroid ligament. This cricothyroid space occupies a trapezoidal area of 3.0 (2.7–3.2) cm^2, and has a 9 (5–12)-mm vertical height[18,19]. Adjacent vascular structures include the

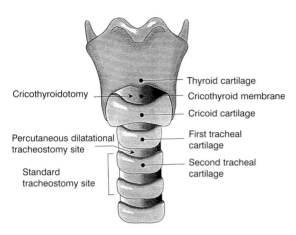

Figure 1 Surgical anatomy of the airway

overlying thyroid isthmus and superior thyroidal artery. The cricoid cartilage is then united with the inferior tracheal cartilage rings by the cricothyroid ligament. Innervation is provided by the superior laryngeal nerve supplying sensory impulses above the vocal cords, and the recurrent laryngeal nerve supplying laryngeal motor and sensory impulses below the vocal cords.

CRICOTHYROIDOTOMY

The modern history of cricothyroidotomy begins with the classic treatise by Chevalier Jackson, whose 30-year experience in treatment of laryngeal stenosis cited 93% of complications occurring with 'high tracheotomy', where 20% involved the cricothyroid cartilage[20]. Therefore, this valuable airway technique was viewed with disfavor until the landmark review of cricothyroidotomy was published by Brantigan and Grow in 1976. They reported only a 6% complication rate in a large case series with no cases of subglottic stenosis described[21].

The indications for cricothyroidotomy are varied and this technique is suitable for both emergency and routine conditions (Table 1). Contraindications are relative, since most

patients are in dire need of airway control and these may include pediatric patients and those with coagulopathy or laryngeal fracture. The procedure itself is simple to perform, but is optimized by meticulous technique.

Procedure

(1) *Position* Neck hyperextension is desirable, using a towel roll beneath the shoulder in the routine setting;

(2) *Stabilization* The non-dominant hand stabilizes the laryngeal cartilage, with the index finger in the superior notch and the thumb and forefinger laterally;

(3) *Cutaneous incision* A vertical incision performed in the midline allows better landmark identification, a greater chance of locating the cricothyroid membrane and less bleeding, but healing is cosmetically inferior to that in the horizontal incision;

(4) *Cricothyroid incision* A horizontal incision inferior to the superior thyroid artery performed as a stab movement, which is carried laterally to the cricoid cartilage and rotated 180° to the opposite cartilage border;

(5) *Stabilization* This requires an assistant with superior and inferior skin hooks to optimize visualization;

(6) *Dilatation* 'Once in, stay in'. The scalpel blade is replaced by a Trousseau dilator or curved hemostat;

(7) *Insertion* A tracheostomy tube (6.0 Fr) is inserted, or, if none is available, an endotracheal tube (ETT) (6.0);

(8) *Confirmation* Assessment of air, suction catheter passage or chest radiograph, noting position, pneumothorax;

(9) *Securing* Stabilization with cloth, tracheal ties, circumferential sutures or tape.

Emergency

The experience with emergency cricothyroidotomy suggests that in selected cases adequate ventilation is achieved, while careful attention to depth and angle of penetration minimizes complications[22]. The procedure is easily and rapidly performed and is the emergency airway procedure of choice, especially in acute airway obstruction[23,24]. The clinical utility of cricothyroidotomy has been demonstrated in those in whom a difficult intubation is encountered.

Prehospital indications for cricothyroidotomy include facial trauma (40%), failed oral intubation (35%) and potential for cervical fracture (5%), with an 88% rate of success[25]. However, in those patients in whom the procedure fails, the outcome is poor – with most patients (80%) in arrest demonstrating poor survival (1.5%) and neurological devastation (66%)[25]. The most common indication for a surgical airway is oromaxillofacial trauma (67%), followed by failed intubation (20%). It is required in 3% of prehospital airway emergencies with a 98% success rate[26].

Patients may also undergo cricothyroidotomy secondary to failed intubation (87%) often due to emesis or hemorrhage (33%), cervical injury (27%), technical failure (21%) and masseter muscle spasm (18%)[27]. The survival rate is 32% with difficulties such as misplacement through the thyrohyoid membrane (33%), insertion time of more than 3 min (26%), unsuccessful procedure (20%), hemorrhage (13%) and thyroid cartilage fracture (7%)[27].

Cricothyroidotomy performed in the trauma setting (7.5%) allowed survival of 59% of the patients, with minor complications occurring in 27%, equivalent to conversion to tracheostomy. Major complications are increased if tracheostomy conversion is required, on the basis of duration of cannulation[28]. Thus, the population associated with emergency cricothyroidotomy is predisposed to poor outcome, because of its time-consuming nature, as the procedure is often instituted late in the course of respiratory failure. Perhaps the adverse outcome may be averted by earlier institution of the procedure in those patient groups profiled.

Routine

The routine indications for cricothyroidotomy include secretion clearance and prolonged mechanical ventilation. Cricothyroidotomy has been recommended for recent sternotomy patients and has a complication rate of 1–9% in patients predisposed by endotracheal intubation of 7 days or longer, a relative contraindication[29]. Clinical experience documented that patients converted from endotracheal intubation to cricothyroidotomy after an average of 7 days, maintained for 59 (3–270) days and decannulated at 38 (6–197) days demonstrated only minimal side-effects: tracheal stenosis and granulation tissue (5%)[30].

This technique has also been explored for management of secretions postoperatively with 72% efficacy, and a complication rate of 3–8% manifested as bleeding. 'Minitracheotomy' through a coniotomy incision had an 87% success rate when maintained for approximately 10 days, enabling effective secretion removal by suction catheter[31]. The standard or emergency cricothyroidotomy may be cannulated with a modified tube to prevent cricoarytenoid disruption, small standard or pediatric tracheostomy tubes (Figure 2). This technique may also be utilized for prolonged management of mechanically ventilated patients, who have been intubated for a short duration (less than 1 week) and are without bleeding diathesis.

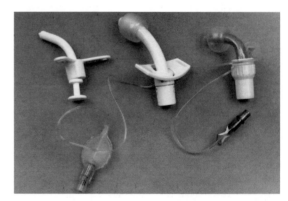

Figure 2 Cricothyroidotomy cannulae. (a) Pediatric uncuffed cannula (Shiley, Irvine, CA), (b) standard tracheostomy cannula 4.0–6.0 (Shiley, Irvine, CA), (c) cricothyroidotomy cannula (Rusch, Kernen, Germany)

Complications

Complications encountered in emergency cricothyroidotomy are often related to massive neck swelling obscuring the thyroid cartilage. These cases are best approached by isolating the hyoid bone located midway between a line from the mental protuberance bisected at half the length of the mandible[32]. The thyroid cartilage and cricothyroid space may be located inferior to the hyoid bone in those with obscured anatomy.

The emergency setting finds complications represented in 18–32% of patients encountered[27,33]. Complications include hemorrhage (5.4%), tube occlusion from debris (5.4%), tube misplacement (4.3%), cartilage fracture (3.6%) and subglottic stenosis (3.6%)[33]. Tube misplacement may occur outside the cricothyroid space in one-third of cases and is found in paratracheal soft tissue or thyroid cartilage, inside the esophagus or positioned retrograde into the pharynx[27,34,35].

Routine cricothyroidotomy allows discussion of long-term complications. The procedure itself is simpler than tracheostomy and is associated with only minimal sequelae: voice change is most common and subglottic stenosis is encountered in rare cases[36]. Patients are predisposed to complications, occurring in half of the cases with cricothyroidotomy for more than 30 days, intubation for more than 7 days, diabetes mellitus and advanced age[37,38]. Another strong correlative is the presence of stomal infection causing granulation tissue and subsequent cartilaginous injury and subsequent stenosis[39]. The procedure is associated with some morbidity (73%) manifested as moderate to severe perichondral inflammation (45%) but with minimal stenosis (0%). Increased mortality (49%) has been isolated as a covariable of patients because of their poor condition[40]. Complications of cricothyroidotomy may also be classified as severe (13%), associated with acute airway difficulty, or major (33%) or non-life threatening but eventually requiring surgery[38]. Major complications occur in 7% and include subglottic stenosis, granulation and tracheomalacia; minor complications occur in 30% and are usually located at the cuff site manifested as ulceration, hemorrhage or abscess[41].

The most sensitive indicator of dysfunction after airway intervention is voice change. This finding is demonstrated in 50–75% of patients and is due to diminished external tensor effect on vocal folds in 48% of cases[42,43]. Also, cricoarytenoid muscle dysfunction occurs by an unknown mechanism with a normal electromyogram (EMG) and muscle biopsy, but is manifested as diminished voice range and lower pitch[44].

The most specific measure of trauma induced by airway intervention is subglottic stenosis. This effect occurs in 4.6% (0–12.5%) of patients[41,43,45,46]. Most modern evaluations suggest that cricothyroidotomy, performed in the appropriate setting without active infection or prolonged intubation, has a decreased rate of subglottic stenosis compared to prolonged endotracheal intubation or tracheostomy.

Percutaneous cricothyroidotomy

The 'cut and poke' cricothyrotomy (using a knife blade with rubber limit and cannulae insertion) was described by Safar and Penninckx in 1967[18]. The 'last ditch' airway was reported in 1979; it is performed with a scalpel blade capable of being carried between two credit cards, and insertion of an intravenous tubing spike connected to positive-pressure ventilation[47].

The first large critical trial utilized the Minitrach (Sims, Keene, NH) system consisting of a 4-mm pediatric ETT placed through a cricothyroid membrane incision made with a guarded knife and introducer. The system was used in the operating room to cannulate patients for up to 45 days, and provided satisfactory therapy for sputum retention in all patients[48]. The Minitrach II system (Sims, Keene, NH, see Figure 3) was re-evaluated as a means of improving pulmonary toilet and demonstrated efficacy, manifested as early discharge from the intensive care unit (ICU) in 88% after limited cannulation for 4 days or less. Postoperatively, minor bleeding (7%) is noted as a side-effect[49]. This method is also recommended in the emergency setting using a high-frequency jet oxygenation delivery system[50]. This apparatus, compared to control, also demonstrated a decrease in postoperative atelectasis on days 1 and 7, while fewer patients required bronchoalveolar lavage for secretion management[51]. Clancy's study, however, cited therapeutic failure in one-third of patients[52] (Figure 4).

The NuTrake system (International Medical Devices, Northridge, CA, see Figure 5) demonstrated more rapid placement and a higher success rate using video instruction to teach trainees[53]. The use of 'minitracheotomy' in 5.9% of cardiothoracic surgery patients, in whom a 20 Fr pediatric tracheostomy tube was placed as a cricothyroidostomy for sputum retention, resulted in a 99% success rate and significant decrease in the need for bronchoscopy[54]. Complications were minimal and only included bleeding (3.5%), since subglottic stenosis was not demonstrated[54]. This procedure has minimal documented mortality, but may be difficult (3%) or impossible (1%) to perform in some patients, owing to cricothyroid calcification[55].

Techniques based on a wire guide may be more amenable to use by practitioners of all specialties. A percutaneous dilatational technique has been described, where needle position and wire guidance are followed by a nasal speculum-like dilator and 6-mm tracheostomy tube. This method, although cumbersome, suggests the use of objects readily available to the critical care physician to cannulate the airway[56]. The Quicktrach device documents prolonged insertion times compared to open technique (83 to 35 s) and a 27% complication rate based on operative experience[57].

The Melker percutaneous dilatational cricothyroidotomy kit (Cook, Bloomington, IN, see Figure 6) allows cricothyroid needle puncture, wire placement and insertion of a unitized anatomically conformed tube and dilator in a single step, minimizing malposition and cartilage damage. This appears to be a safe and effective technique. Prior cricothyroidotomy devices have an associated difficulty of insertion (54%) and can result in mediastinal puncture, paratracheal cannula placement and

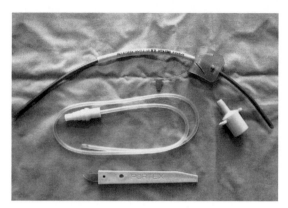

Figure 3 Minitrach II system (Sims, Keene, NH)

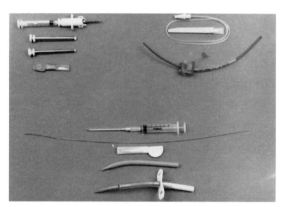

Figure 4 Percutaneous cricothyroidotomy. (a) NuTrake (International Medical Devices, Northridge, CA), (b) Minitrach II (Sims, Keene, NH), (c) percutaneous cricothyroidotomy kit (Cook, Bloomington, IN)

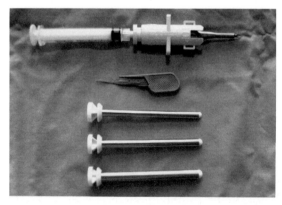

Figure 5 NuTrake system (International Medical Devices, Northridge, CA)

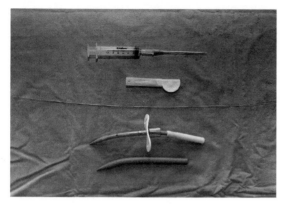

Figure 6 Percutaneous dilatational cricothyroid-otomy kit (Cook, Bloomington, IN)

subcutaneous emphysema, making subsequent airway maneuvers even more difficult[58].

Correct position is verified ideally by fiberoptic bronchoscopy, but suction catheter passage described in 11% of cases, air flow or end-tidal CO_2 detection may suffice[58]. Percutaneous cricothyroidotomy, a modified surgical technique, allows placement of a definitive airway in the routine or emergency setting by practitioners of all specialties. However, the procedure may result in significant complications in those patients with anatomic distortion or bleeding diathesis, or when placed by the inexperienced operator, but it should be included in the practitioner's airway repertoire.

PERCUTANEOUS TRANSLARYNGEAL VENTILATION

The historical development of this airway intervention was directed by an environment where there was no good solution for a failed airway, since cricothyroidotomy was not recommended, owing to subglottic stenosis during the early period, and tracheostomy was not an emergency procedure. Transtracheal artificial respiration was described by Reed and coworkers in 1954 in a canine model using a tapered 13-gauge steel needle and a 15-l/min flow system for 30 min[59]. This system allowed adequate oxygenation (15.7 to 19.2 vol%), but inadequate ventilation with hypercarbia (CO_2

38–103 mmHg) and resultant respiratory acidosis (pH 7.45–7.08), causing hemodynamic depression with a decreased mean arterial pressure and heart rate, and increased central venous pressure[59].

The pressure–flow characteristics of resuscitation needles were analyzed and the 13-gauge needle with 88 cmH_2O pressure generated 200 ml/s gas flow[60]. The normal adult has a peak flow of 400 ml/s and this system was only capable of maintaining adequate ventilation in a complete obstruction model for slightly longer than breath holding (86–71 s)[60]. This method was further explored, and it was concluded that the 18- and 16-gauge catheters were unacceptable as ventilation tools with survival of 5 and 15 min, respectively[9]. The 13-gauge system allows survival to 60 min in dogs, but in a calf model more analogous to humans, survival was achieved for only 16 min[9]. Thus, this current technology is limited by cannula size of 14-gauge or larger at the current flow rates and O_2 delivery systems.

Transtracheal ventilation is indicated for failed intubation with operator comfort, or as the procedure of choice in partial airway obstruction. There are few contraindications to the procedure except operator inexperience, laryngeal trauma, coagulopathy or perhaps complete airway obstruction (Table 1).

Procedure

(1) *Position* Neck extension if no cervical trauma;

(2) *Stabilization* Non-dominant hand on thyroid cartilage;

(3) *Palpation* Index finger guide to cricothyroid membrane;

(4) *Apparatus* Saline-filled syringe, catheter over needle assembly, connector and oxygen source (50 psi);

(5) *Entry* Catheter-syringe directed at 45° caudad to avoid posterior tracheal wall until free flow of air is obtained;

(6) *Connection* Withdrawal of stylet; tubing from oxygen source (50 psi) connected;

(7) *Ventilation*   Ratio of inspiration (1) : expiration (4) seconds to prevent air trapping;

(8) *Stabilization*   Control of catheter always retained until it is secured in the neck by more permanent means;

(9) *Monitoring*   Evidence of barotrauma–hypotension, subcutaneous emphysema;

(10) *Confirmation*   Chest radiograph: position, pneumothorax.

Mechanics

The most critical issue regarding efficacy of ventilation is the diameter of the catheter, where flow varies inversely with the radius to the fourth power according to the Law of Poiseuille. The minimum catheter size should be 14-gauge (235 ml/s), which demonstrates a ten-fold flow increase compared to a 22-gauge catheter (26 ml/s) and is available in most institutions[61]. Specifically, a 12-gauge catheter (area 6.15 mm^2) compares favorably to a 3.0-mm ETT (area 7.06 mm^2), which allows ventilation at lower pressure settings[62].

The catheter design is also significant. The curved Tuohy needle deflects the oxygen flow parallel to the long axis of the trachea, resulting in a two-fold flow increase, decreased barotrauma and improved oxygenation and ventilation[63]. An anatomically S-shaped catheter has also proved superior in stability and ventilation, owing to its large tidal volume, and decreased incidence of posterior wall perforation[64].

The flow delivery system is next in importance when determining ventilatory efficacy. The minimum pressure gradient required to generate flow through a small-diameter cannula is 0.1–0.5 psi (7–35 cmH$_2$O), which is achieved by precise control of the inspiratory time of the system with 50 psi (3420 cmH$_2$O)[62]. The pressure gradient required to achieve adequate ventilation is provided only by a jet source of 50 psi, not a bag-valve-mask or demand-valve system generating less than 60 cmH$_2$O of pressure[65]. A previously described model using a 14-gauge cannula found a five-fold increase in

flow (235–1034 ml/s), enough to achieve adequate ventilation by the substitution of a jet system of 50 psi compared to bag valve mask ventilation[61].

Clearly, the lower-flow 15-l/min systems may provide adequate oxygenation, but they provide inadequate ventilation with survival limited to 1–2 h before patients are affected by hypercarbia and respiratory acidosis[66–69]. The flow delivery system used for long-term jet ventilation is more sophisticated. The high-frequency oscillation (HFO) system provides ventilatory rates of 400–2400/min delivered in a sinusoidal pattern, while high-frequency jet ventilation (HFJV) is deliverable at rates of 110–400/min and high-frequency positive-pressure ventilation (HFPPV) at rates of 60–110/min; this system uses a square wave, where frequency affects the linear nature of flow[70,71]. Ventilation at high frequency is best interpreted by principles of fluid rather than gas mechanics. Ventilation efficacy and barotrauma are optimized by central columnal flow as opposed to eccentric airflow[72]. The flow viscosity is reduced by adequate humidity, further improving ventilation[73].

Parameters that may be altered to affect ventilation include tidal volume, which results in a 67–95% variance in CO_2 elimination with alveolar ventilation proportional to the square root of tidal volume[74,75]. Altering the frequency results in a smaller CO_2 variance (0.1–14%)[74]. Increasing frequency from low (1 Hz, 60/min) to high (5 Hz, 300/min) increases CO_2 clearance by decreasing dead space and increasing alveolar ventilation[75,76]. The net change in CO_2 clearance is minimally affected by frequency alteration compared to other modalities[77]. The addition of excess positive end-expiratory pressure (PEEP) may paradoxically decrease alveolar ventilation[74]. However, the appropriate level of PEEP ranging from 0 to 1.0 kPa may preserve arterial O_2 tension without an increase in shunt or adverse hemodynamic effects[78].

Prolonging the inspiratory/expiratory time ratio from 0.25 to 1.0 increases alveolar ventilation in an efficient fashion, but may cause myocardial depression secondary to decreased preload and cardiac index[77,79]. These alterations may cause an increase in mean and peak airway pressure with impaired ventilation[77,80]. This effect may become detrimental by decreasing venous return, and it may be counteracted by volume loading to preserve mean arterial pressure and cardiac output[81]. Thus, the patient can benefit from the increased driving pressure resulting in improved ventilation[82].

Clinical findings

The percutaneous transtracheal ventilation system was described as a resuscitation adjunct in 80 patients treated at the accident site, with even a truck tire theoretically suggested for use as the source of compressed air (50 psi) as a bridge to tracheostomy[83]. A canine hemorrhagic shock model demonstrated equivalent oxygenation (PO_2 322 mmHg), ventilation (PCO_2 21 mmHg) and acidosis (pH 7.14) comparing the percutaneous transtracheal ventilation and standard ETT systems[84]. The indication for emergency use includes the presence of partial airway obstruction. If this obstruction is due to a laryngotracheal foreign body, then percutaneous transtracheal ventilation may assist with expelling the object[85].

Although potentially contraindicated, use in complete airway obstruction models suggests that low-flow delivery provides adequate oxygenation, while suboptimal ventilation allows CO_2 to accumulate to prohibitive levels (PCO_2 256 mmHg) curtailing use at 1.5 h[86]. Barotrauma becomes a concern in complete obstruction, and a double-lumen cannula, permitted hypercapnia, decreased minute ventilation and prolonged inspiratory/expiratory time ratio have been recommended to allow CO_2 egress[87]. Partial obstruction finds ventilation adequate to supernormal, as it progresses from 40% to 80% and a respiratory alkalosis is developed[88]. The last issue is the use of percutaneous transtracheal ventilation for a controlled airway leak, as opposed to laryngeal disruption, where this technique may be contraindicated. A canine tracheal trauma model with a 1 × 1 cm window suggests that percutaneous transtracheal ventilation provides adequate ventilation with a minimal controlled leak to maintain adequate respiration[89].

Percutaneous transtracheal ventilation has been used for emergency (46%) and routine (24%) airway obstruction with reasonable success, but with complications encountered such as catheter displacement, total expiratory obstruction and barotrauma[90]. This technique has also been explored for difficult intubation with no adverse effects, morbidity or mortality[91]. This device has proven more effective in providing adequate oxygenation in 71% of cases than ventilation (0%)[92]. Clinical evaluations have used the Arrow Emergency Infusion Device (Arrow International, Reading, PA), an intravenous 8.5 Fr catheter, to provide adequate ventilation in partial complete obstruction models[93]. The device, a 13-gauge angulated catheter with side holes, is placed through the cricothyroid space or intratracheal cartilage connected via a 15-mm male adapter with Luer lock fitting and stabilized with Velcro wrap, and has been used successfully in patients[94]. The Minitrach II system (Sims, Keene, NH), a cricothyroidostomy tube, has been adapted for jet ventilation proving 94% efficacious[95] (Figure 7).

Complications

The airway inflammation associated with ultra-high-frequency jet ventilation (250–400/min)

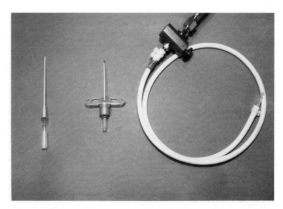

Figure 7 Percutaneous translaryngeal ventilation apparatus. (a) Catheter (Deseret, Sandy, UT), (b) transcricothyrotomy device (VBM Medizintechnik, Sulz/Neckar, West Germany), (c) jet (50 psi) system

occurs in 100% of cases manifested as erosion, necrosis and leukocyte infiltration at the catheter tip and is greater than with conventional high-frequency (150/min) and conventional ventilation (20/min)[96]. However, others have reported an equivalent frequency of laryngotracheomalacia and vocal cord scarring from percutaneous transtracheal ventilation and conventional ventilation[97]. Endolaryngeal subglottic hemorrhage may occur secondary to catheter trauma of the perforating branch of the cricothyroid artery or vein, as well as posterior tracheal wall perforation[98].

Cardiac sequelae are related to the presence of air trapping often caused by increased PEEP. Increasing PEEP is productive to a point with improved peak pressure, mean arterial pressures (PaO$_2$ 104–194 mmHg) and shunt fraction (0.45% to 0.20%)[98]. This PEEP becomes limiting usually at a level over 20 cmH$_2$O causing myocardial depression and increased intracranial pressure[99]. The hypovolemic patient finds adverse cardiac effects minimized by maintenance of lower-frequency ventilation (100 vs. 200/min)[100].

The pulmonary complications of percutaneous transtracheal ventilation include barotrauma manifested as pneumothorax – unilateral or bilateral – pneumomediastinum and subcutaneous emphysema[101–104]. This barotrauma may also be transmitted to the abdominal cavity, resulting in pneumoperitoneum and hypotension by catheter impingement against the tracheal wall[101,105]. However, one of the benefits of percutaneous transtracheal ventilation is a decreased rate of aspiration compared to conventional cuffed ETT or head of bed elevation (30–45°) recommendations[106].

Miscellaneous side-effects of percutaneous transtracheal ventilation include an increased intracranial pressure due to decreased cerebral elastance[99]. This effect is also related to elevated peak airway pressures, where there is a decreased cerebral venous outflow increasing intracranial pressure, which is lessened in HFJV compared to conventional ventilation[107]. The renal effects of HFJV are related to excess PEEP where, although the stroke and cardiac indices are improved, the plasma renin activity is increased, causing decreased urinary flow, creatinine clearance and fractional excretion of sodium[108]. Thus, percutaneous transtracheal ventilation is a safe and effective airway intervention in the appropriate setting, which includes absence of laryngeal pathology, coagulopathy and total airway obstruction. Conventional manual ventilation with a jet (50 psi) O$_2$ source is limited by ventilation (1–2 h), while oxygenation is adequate. This ventilation efficiency may be improved, allowing longer-term support by a high-frequency (100–400/min, 1.7–6.7 Hz) ventilation system.

TRACHEOSTOMY

Vesalius in 1555 published a compendium illustrating a tracheostomy performed on a sow by cherubs, hinting at potential complications of the procedure itself. His description of tracheal dissection includes the issue of recurrent laryngeal nerve injury and reads 'but that life may in a manner of speaking be restored to the animal, an opening must be attempted in the trunk of the trachea; into which a reed or cane should be put; you will then blow into this; so that the lung may rise again and the animal takes in air'[109].

This technique again resurfaced in the diphtheria epidemic of the 19th century where Trousseau described its use to prevent asphyxia and obstruction. Jackson's classic treatise discussed the tracheotomic causes of laryngeal stenosis in 1921, specifically a hasty operation, general anesthesia, 'high tracheotomy', cricoid cartilage division, wound suture closure, poor postoperative care, cannulae of improper size, shape and material or having fenestrations, and neglect of ordering decent cleanliness in weaning off the cannulae[20]. The most well-described complication in diphtheria survivors was subglottic stenosis (6.5%). 'The difficulties and dangers; experienced in so many cases on attempting after the pulmonary disease had subsided, a removal of the canula (sic) from the trachea in which it has remained for some time is well known in many. Chief among these are the sudden attacks of asphyxia, etc., which occur at this period'[110].

Indications

The indications for tracheostomy are diverse and the only contraindication is the necessity for an emergency airway, since this procedure is time consuming and requires surgical expertise. Comparison of emergency versus routine tracheostomy finds a two-fold complication rate due to time spent for isolation of the trachea because of resultant bleeding[111]. The procedure requires more attention to detail and is truly an operative intervention, usually performed in the operating suite followed by the ICU or critical care unit if conditions warrant[112].

Procedure

(1) *Setting*   Operative suite or intensive care unit;

(2) *Position*   Head and neck extended;

(3) *Anesthesia*   Local preferable (lidocaine, epinephrine) over general anesthesia for the unstable patient;

(4) *Skin incision*   Transverse incision 1 cm above the sternal notch and 2 cm below the cricoid cartilage in the triangle formed by the medial sternocleidomastoid and cricoid cartilage;

(5) *Subcutaneous*   Sharp dissection to identify fascial planes;

(6) *Fascia*   Division of strap muscles in midline;

(7) *Neurovascular*   The midline approach avoids anterior jugular vein and recurrent laryngeal nerve;

(8) *Thyroid isthmus*   Retraction superiorly and transection with suture ligature instead of cautery. If not divided, occlusion can occur with decannulation;

(9) *Tracheal incision*   Local anesthesia. Site: 2nd–3rd, 3rd–4th tracheal rings, incision not stab method. Transverse incision in intramembranous portion of tracheal ring;

(10) *Tracheal resection*   Incision design – vertical, horizontal, flap, tracheal window;

(11) *Stabilization*   Skin hooks or Allis clamp: superior–inferior;

(12) *Anastomosis*   Exteriorize: tracheal flap to skin. Stay suture: lateral trachea to skin;

(13) *Cannulation*   Tube 50–75% diameter of trachea. Insertion at right angle, rotation caudad. Sizing: male (6–10 Fr), female (4–8 Fr);

(14) *Confirmation*   Air flow, suction catheter, radiography;

(15) *Securing*   Tracheal ties on suture;

(16) *Closure*   Loosely approximated to prevent subcutaneous emphysema.

Design

Tracheostomy success and complications are dependent on surgical design and equipment used. The most stable approach may include opposing U-shaped flaps, superior and inferior, from the anterior tracheal wall to the suprasternal notch; this has proven to be well tolerated, efficient and reversible[113]. A single inverted-U flap has been explored in a canine model featuring less distortion of the tracheal lumen, stoma site patency and better healing[114]. The oval tracheal window with a diameter one-half of the tracheal width has been suggested as optimal placement due to vascular anastomosis with both horizontal and vertical components[115]. These methods, compared clinically, suggest that the lowest rate of stenosis occurs with the vertical (35%) incision followed by the horizontal H (37%), and that the most significant occurs with the inferior trapdoor (49%)[116].

The design characteristics of the tracheostomy tube are significant. Pressure necrosis occurring between the posterior trachea and vertical body at the thoracic inlet may be minimized by shape – modification of length and curvature as well as good, stable fixation[117] (Figure 8). Longer tracheostomy tubes may impact against the carina or result in a right mainstem intubation[118]. Thus, the tracheostomy tube should be kept soft but resilient, resist torque and be of the appropriate length (Table 2) (Figure 9).

The fenestrated tube allows the patient's use of the upper airway for speech and better respiratory toilet but is positioned with the fenestration required to be between the superior and inferior tracheal margins[119]. This fenestration is often associated with obstruction, so individualizing its placement, as well as using multiple small fenestrations compared to one large fenestration are advantageous[120] (Figure 10).

The ideal tracheostomy cuff should have a longer intratracheal distance with a large surface area and be of the high-volume, low-pressure variety[121,122]. The cuff shape associated with a decrease in complications is a pear-shaped, mobile variant opposed to a spherical fixed segment[123]. The last issue includes cuff pressure regulation (maximum 3 kPa) instituted for moderate-term ventilation,

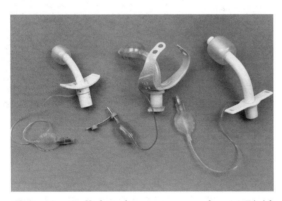

Figure 8 Cuffed tracheostomy cannulae. (a) Rigid composition (Shiley, Irvine, CA), (b) soft composition (Sims, Keene, NH), (c) soft composition (Shiley, Irvine, CA)

resulting in only 5% tracheal damage[123]. Prevention of cuff complications is best addressed by cuff inflation to audible leak pressure, followed by alternating the cuff sites or hourly cuff deflation[124] (Figure 11).

Emergency

The emergency indications for tracheostomy are few but occur when endotracheal intubation is impossible, and cricothyroidotomy is precluded by high-grade upper airway obstruction, massive neck swelling or laryngeal fracture. When these conditions are encountered, a finder needle saline syringe system is helpful in locating the trachea[125].

Routine

Tracheostomy has an associated morbidity (47%), mainly pneumonia, and mortality (6%) often found with delayed hemorrhage in those with prolonged intubation[126]. The mortality in ICU patients alone (46%) warrants that their disease condition be delineated from that due to the procedure itself[13].

This issue assumes importance when discussing the location where tracheostomy is performed. Bedside tracheostomy may be associated with minimal mortality (0%) and morbidity (6%), where complications such as bleeding or pneumothorax present early (5%; within 2 days) rather than late (1%; after 2 days), when infection mainly occurs[127]. This procedure has been performed at the bedside safely in selected patient populations under local and intravenous sedation without

Table 2 Tracheostomy tube size

Tracheostomy tube size	Inner diameter (mm)	Outer diameter (mm)	Cuffed, single cannula length (mm)
4	4.0	8.5	55–67
5	5.0	7.0	—
6	6.0	8.1–8.3	75–78
7	7.0	9.6–9.7	82
8	8.0	10.9–11.0	84–87
9	9.0	12.1	—
10	10.0	13.3–13.5	84–98

complications and avoiding the risk of operating-room transfer[128]. Timing strategies for tracheostomy are numerous and should not be arbitrary, but individualized to the particular patient.

One clinical trial examined tracheostomy performed in burn patients on day 1 (7%), day 8 (17%) and day 14 (58%), and maintained for 33 days without clear correlation with complications[129]. Early tracheostomy (4 days) has been recommended in trauma patients, resulting in a decreased ventilation requirement due to less pneumonia, allowing an earlier wean[130]. Similarly, early tracheostomy (7 days) has proven superior, shown by a decrease in mortality (0%), morbidity (40%), mechanical ventilation, length of hospital stay and ICU stay[131]. However, in a study of trauma patients, of interest because of rigid head posture and hard cervical collar, there was no difference in laryngotracheal complications between early (less than 2 weeks) and late (more than 2 weeks) tracheostomy[132].

Current recommendations are based on clinical evaluation. There are isolated data to suggest that nasal intubation is equivalent to tracheostomy in the incidence and onset of complications[133]. Endotracheal intubation may be superior to tracheostomy in specific patient populations such as those with burns, or those with an increased incidence of granuloma (29%) and stenosis (23%)[134]. The preponderance of evidence suggests that tracheostomy (14%) is associated with less laryngotracheal trauma than nasal or orotracheal intubation (57%)[135,136]. Also, patients find tracheostomy more comfortable, as it allows them to communicate effectively and simplifies nursing airway care; 92% of patients prefer this technique for ETT requirements of more than 10 days[136].

Complications

Most initial perioperative tracheostomy complications are minor, including hemorrhage or subcutaneous emphysema (2.4%), and the incidence of major early complications such as loss of airway control, obstruction or excessive blood loss (0%) is minimal[137]. The overall

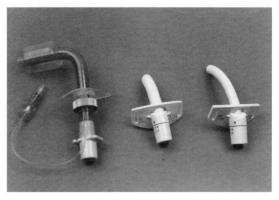

Figure 9 Tracheostomy variable length and cuff. (a) Variable length (Rusch, Kernen, Germany), (b) laryngectomy (Shiley, Irvine, CA), (c) cuffless (Shiley, Irvine, CA)

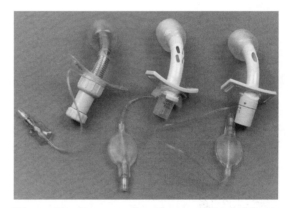

Figure 10 Fenestrated tracheostomy cannulae. (a) Single, soft (Rusch, Kernen, Germany), (b) multiple (Shiley, Irvine, CA), (c) single (Shiley, Irvine, CA)

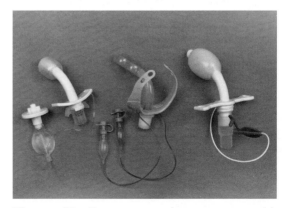

Figure 11 Pressure regulator systems. (a) Pressure release (Shiley, Irvine, CA), (b) double-cuff (Sims, Keene, NH), (c) foam-cuff (Bivona, Gary, IN)

complication rate of tracheostomy is 28.5% (6–48%), which is less than that encountered in endotracheal intubation[132,137–139] (Table 3).

The most frequently discussed condition is subglottic stenosis. The lesion is found at the cuff site, where intracuff pressure may translate into tracheal wall pressures of 35–214 mmHg causing circumferential ulceration, pressure necrosis and subsequent scarring[140,141]. The incidence of this complication has decreased from 6% in the 19th century to 1% (0.9–2.4%) today[13,110,138,142]. These lesions may occur at the stoma or cuff site, and they have a distinct pathogenesis and outcome[143].

Perhaps the most common complication, however, is infection with far-reaching sequelae. Those with tracheostomy have a higher rate of lower respiratory tract colonization (76%) with Gram-negative rods, such as *Pseudomonas aeruginosa*, often progressing to tracheobronchitis[144]. The bacteria that colonized the respiratory tree in those with tracheostomy are increased in their number and their adherence properties[145]. More severe infections include necrotizing tracheitis associated with purulent peristomal drainage (100%), causing difficulty with ventilation – air leak and stomal cavitation (66%)[146].

Patients are predisposed to this condition by colonization with *Pseudomonas*, *Enterobacter*

Table 3 Complications associated with tracheostomy. From references 8, 13, 137–139, 146–148, 150, 151, 154, 171

	Incidence (%)
Common	
Pneumonia	22
Tracheobronchitis	8
Hemorrhage	8
Stomal infection	3
Tracheoinnominate fistulae	3
Subcutaneous emphysema	2
Subglottic stenosis	0.9
Granulation	0.8
Tracheoarterial hemorrhage	0.7
Rare	
Necrotizing tracheitis	
Paratracheal abscess	
Posterior wall laceration	
Tracheoesophageal fistula	
Mediastinal emphysema	

or *Klebsiella*, suture fixation, neurological injury and tight closure of the incision. Infection is treated by topical or systemic antibiotics, or use of a Montgomery Silastic T-tube stent[146]. Paratracheal mediastinal abscess has been described and is associated with upper lobe consolidation and septicemia[147]. Tracheal soft tissue injury is localized to the posterior wall in cases of mucosal rigidity associated with radiation therapy or infection and results in poor ventilation after tube insertion[148]. Massive dissecting emphysema can occur when the tracheostomy tube is malpositioned in the pretracheal fascia and positive-pressure ventilation is applied[149].

Life-threatening hemorrhage involving the brachiocephalic trunk occurs in 0.6–1.1% of patients owing to anterior cuff erosion[150,151]. Trachea–innominate hemorrhage occurs in the setting of cuff overdistension, low-lying tracheostomy and anterior soft tissue damage caused by polymicrobial stomal sepsis, with outcome based on control of the brachiocephalic trunk[151–153]. Acute hemostasis is achieved by cuff hyperinflation, oral intubation, periostomal anterior digital pressure or ligature of the innominate artery and brachiocephalic trunk resection or reconstruction with autogenous venous graft, and is associated with good neurological outcome[150,152].

Abnormal vascular erosion may also present as a fistula. Common carotid artery involvement can be produced by a metal cannula and often occurs during the wound healing phase after tumor resection, occurring in 2.6% of patients[154]. Trachea–innominate fistulae occur in the extratracheal position at the tracheostomy tube elbow, while the intratracheal portion is caused by the tube tip or cuff[155]. Patients are predisposed by low-lying tracheostomy (below the fourth tracheal ring), high innominate artery position, inflammation or steroid use[155]. Thus, trachea–innominate hemorrhage can result in exsanguination and hemodynamic instability, while trachea–innominate fistulae present with airway obstruction and asphyxia, with qualitatively less bleeding found (100–150 ml)[156].

Tracheoesophageal fistulae occasionally occur secondarily to compression between an overdistended cuff and rigid nasogastric tube presenting as aspiration. They are treated conservatively with drainage in a single-stage repair[157].

Assessment and therapy

The institution of tracheostomy requires constant vigilance and routine assessment of complications. The institution of a prophylactic examination has demonstrated miscellaneous difficulties in 17%, asymptomatic stomal size narrowing (16%) and bleeding (10%) severe enough to require tracheal resection in 8% of patients[158]. The standard of care includes routine bronchoscopic surveillance weekly to monthly as necessary[159]. This video technique is especially helpful in the diagnosis of phonation difficulty (66%) and aspiration (46%), delineating peripheral nerve or central cord dysfunction[160]. Laryngeal tomography has been replaced by computed tomography in the diagnosis of glottic abnormalities[161]. The need for therapeutic intervention for subglottic stenosis may be due to the higher likelihood of survival with current resuscitation techniques[162]. Patients are predisposed by abnormal neck position (48%), low-lying tracheostomy or aesthenic habitus with damage most often occurring at the cannula tip (67%)[163].

Medical therapy includes the use of topical and systemic antibiotics, since stenosis is related to the acute inflammatory infectious phase[164]. The use of systemic corticosteroids has been explored to address the reactive scarring phase[161]. Progressive balloon dilatation (28–38 Fr) has been described for this condition[165]. Surgical repair begins with planning, and is required for patients with more than 50% tracheal narrowing[166]. Laryngotracheal cicatricial stenosis occurs most commonly at the cricoid cartilage (50%), requiring transverse partial resection with a manubrium sterni bone graft often required[167]. Tracheal stenosis most often results from endotracheal trauma (74%), causing severe stenosis (80%) with >1 cm narrowing (56%)[168]. The surgical approach includes primary resection with end-to-end anastomosis or multistage construction using endothesis[162,168].

Percutaneous tracheostomy

Percutaneous tracheostomy using a large-bore needle and wire guide was described in 1976, possibly for emergency use[169]. Current discussion centers on the use of this technique in the ICU at the bedside. This percutaneous tracheostomy technique has been used for excessive secretions (51%), prolonged intubation (37%) or neurological dysfunction (25%), and is performed electively (77%), urgently (28%) or in an emergency (5%)[170]. This technique was successful in 90% of patients when performed in the emergency department, 70% in the ICU or 46% in the operating room, with minimal morbidity (4.9%), but a single intraoperative death (1%) has been described[170].

Procedure

(1) *Position* Neck hyperextension;

(2) *Anesthesia* Local preferable (lidocaine with epinephrine);

(3) *Landmarks* Horizontal incision (2 cm midway between cricothyroid membrane and sternal notch in midline);

(4) *Puncture* Between tracheal ring 1,2 intramembranous portion punctured at 45° caudad angle avoiding posterior tracheal wall;

(5) *Aspiration* Intratracheal position confirmed by aspiration of air through a saline-filled syringe;

(6) *Catheter* Catheter advanced over needle, air aspiration reconfirmation;

(7) *Guidewire* Wire inserted and catheter removed;

(8) *Dilatation* Passage of progressively larger dilators;

(9) *Tracheostomy tube* Tube passed with largest dilator subsequently removed;

(10) *Confirmation* Position confirmed by air entry and suction catheter passage;

(11) *Stabilization* Tracheal ties or suture.

Modification of this technique includes the Rapitrach system that has a hinged tool dilator demonstrating safe, effective placement[171,172]. The NuTrake (International Medical Device, Northridge, CA) system using a steel cannula has been used for both percutaneous cricothyroidotomy and tracheostomy. The original progressive dilator technique was described by Ciaglia and co-workers in 1985 and stressed entry between the cricoid cartilage and first tracheal ring to reduce the incidence and severity of complications (0%)[173]. A clinical trial comparing the Rapitrach (Premier Medical, Norristown, PA) and Cook (Bloomington, IN) devices and conventional tracheostomy demonstrated procedure times of 5, 15 and 60 min, respectively[174]. However, the highest complication rate was found in the Rapitrach system[151]. The Cook device offers an appropriate compromise in the rapidity of the technique and minimal complication rate, especially with bronchoscopic guidance (Figure 12).

The success of the percutaneous tracheostomy procedure involves appropriate patient selection with a failure rate of 22% in those with 'non-ideal anatomy'[175]. The best of circumstances allows the procedure to be performed in 30 s instead of 3 min for standard tracheostomy[176]. The procedure has a 94% success rate with failure cited when performed by non-surgeons due to poor visualization for bleeding[177,178]. The postoperative result has been optimal (95%) with decannulation possible in up to 100% of patients[170,179].

The complication rate is minimal for 4% (0–14%) and mortality has been cited at 1%[170,176,179,180]. The complication rate of 4% in the percutaneous technique, mainly hemorrhage, compares favorably to that of the

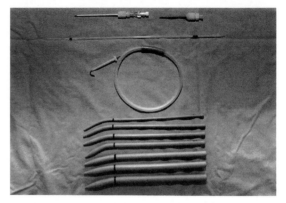

Figure 12 Percutaneous device. Ciaglia percutaneous tracheostomy system (Cook, Bloomington, IN)

standard procedure (18%) where obstruction, hemorrhage, pneumothorax and wound infection figure prominently[181]. However, several cases of life-threatening hemorrhage have been reported with the percutaneous technique, as has pneumothorax[182,183]. Laryngeal tomography confirms the advantage of percutaneous versus standard tracheostomy with decreased overall complications (25% vs. 58%), especially events associated with predecannulation (in 13% vs. 46%) and postdecannulation (27% vs. 88%)[184]. The incidence of complications may be minimized by endoscopic guidance of the percutaneous technique, confirming intratracheal placement and guiding insertion of the tracheostomy tube[185,186].

CONCLUSION

The practitioner attempting endotracheal intubation should in all cases be prepared to attempt a surgical airway – percutaneous jet ventilation, cricothyroidotomy or, in selected patients, tracheostomy in case of failure. The particular technique should vary with operator experience and the clinical setting (emergency or routine), and be individualized to each patient encountered.

References

1. Redan JA, Livingston DH, Tortella BJ, *et al*. The value of intubating and paralyzing patients with suspected head injury in the emergency department. *J Trauma* 1991;31:371–5

2. Murphy-Macabobby M, Marshall WJ, Schneider C, *et al*. Neuromuscular blockade in aeromedical airway management. *Ann Emerg Med* 1992;21:664–8

3. Roberts DJ, Clinton JE, Ruiz E. Neuromuscular blockade for critical patients in the emergency department. *Ann Emerg Med* 1986;15:152–6

4. Ligier B, Buchman TG, Breslow MJ, *et al*. The role of anesthetic induction agents and neuromuscular blockade in the endotracheal intubation of trauma victims. *Surg Gynecol Obstet* 1991;173:477–81

5. O'Brien DJ, Danzl DF, Hooker EA, *et al*. Prehospital blind nasotracheal intubation by paramedics. *Ann Emerg Med* 1989;18:612–17

6. Suderman VS, Crosby ET, Lui A. Elective oral tracheal intubation in cervical spine-injured adults. *Can J Anaesth* 1991;38:785–9

7. Meschino A, Devitt JH, Koch JP, *et al*. The safety of awake tracheal intubation in cervical spine injury. *Can J Anaesth* 1992;39:114–17

8. Holley J, Jorden R. Airway management in patients with unstable cervical spine fractures. *Ann Emerg Med* 1989;18:1237–9

9. Hughes RK. Needle tracheostomy. *Arch Surg* 1966;93:834–7

10. Bivens HG, Ford S, Bezmalinovic Z. The effect of axial traction during orotracheal intubation of the trauma victim with an unstable cervical spine. *Ann Emerg Med* 1988;17:25–9

11. Bishop MJ, Harrington RM, Tencer AF. Force applied during tracheal intubation. *Anesth Analg* 1992;74:411–14

12. Majernick TG, Bieniek R, Houston JB, *et al*. Cervical spine movement during orotracheal intubation. *Ann Emerg Med* 1986;15:417–20

13. Minard G, Kudsk KA, Croce MA. Laryngotracheal trauma. *Am Surg* 1992;58:181–7

14. Sosis MB. What is the safest endotracheal tube for Nd-YAG laser surgery? A comparative study. *Anesth Analg* 1989;69:802–4

15. Lambert GE Jr, McMurry GT. Laryngotracheal trauma: recognition and management. *J Am Coll Emerg Physicians* 1976;5:883–7

16. Steinert R, Lullwit E. Failed intubation with case reports. *Halls Nasen Ohrenheilkund* 1987;35:439–42

17. Goldberg J, Levy PS, Morkovin V, *et al*. Mortality from traumatic injuries. A case–control study using data from the National Hospital Discharge survey. *Med Care* 1983;21:692–704

18. Safar P, Penninckx J. Cricothyroid membrane with special cannula. *Anesthesiology* 1967;28:943–8

19. Caparosa RJ, Zabatsky AR. Practical aspects of the cricothyroid space. *Laryngoscope* 1959;67:577

20. Jackson C. High tracheotomy and other errors the chief causes of chronic laryngeal stenosis. *Surg Gynecol Obstet* 1921;32:392–8

21. Brantigan CO, Grow JB Sr. Cricothyroidotomy: elective use in respirator problems requiring tracheotomy. *J Thorac Cardiovasc Surg* 1976;71:72–81

22. Weiss S. A new emergency cricothyroidotomy instrument. *J Trauma* 1983;23:155–8

23. McDowell DE. Cricothyroidostomy for airway access. *South Med J* 1982;75:282–4

24. Plummer WB. The cricothyroidotomy – a lifesaving adjunct in acute obstructive asphyxia. *J Georgia Dent Assoc* 1969;43:35–8

25. Spaite DW, Joseph M. Prehospital cricothyrotomy: an investigation of indications, technique, complications, and patient outcome. *Ann Emerg Med* 1990;19:279–85

26. Boyle MF, Hatton D, Sheets C. Surgical cricothyrotomy performed by air ambulance flight nurses: A 5-year experience. *J Emerg Med* 1993;11:41–5

27. McGill J, Clinton JE, Ruiz E. Cricothyrotomy in the emergency department. *Ann Emerg Med* 1982;11:361–4

28. DeLaurier GA, Hawkins ML, Treat RC, *et al*. Acute airway management. Role of cricothyroidotomy. *Am Surg* 1990;56:12–15

29. Boyd AD, Romita MC, Conlan AA, *et al*. A clinical evaluation of cricothyroidotomy. *Surg Gynecol Obstet* 1979;149:365–8

30. O'Connor JV, Reddy K, Ergin MA, *et al*. Minitracheotomy for prolonged ventilatory support after cardiac operations. *Ann Thorac Surg* 1985;39:353–4

31. Pedersen J, Schurizek BA, Melson NC, *et al*. Minitracheotomy in the treatment of postoperative sputum retention and atelectasis. *Acta Anaesthesiol Scand* 1988;32:426–8

32. Simon RR, Brenner BE. Emergency cricothyroidotomy in the patient with massive neck swelling: Part 1: Anatomical aspects. *Crit Care Med* 1983;11:114–18

33. Nugent WL, Rhee KJ, Wisner DH. Can nurses perform surgical cricothyrotomy with acceptable success and complication rates? *Ann Emerg Med* 1991;20:367–70

34. Slobodkin D, Topliff S, Raife JH. Retrograde intubation of the pharynx: an unusual

complication of emergency cricothyrotomy. *Ann Emerg Med* 1992;21:220–2

35. Ryan DW, Dark JH, Misra U, *et al.* Intra-oesophageal placement of minitracheotomy tube. *Intensive Care Med* 1989;15:538–9

36. Holst M, Hedenstierna G, Kumlien JA, *et al.* Five years experience of coniotomy. *Intensive Care Med* 1985;11:202–6

37. Kuriloff DB, Setzen M, Portnoy W. Laryngotracheal injury following cricothy-roidotomy. *Laryngoscope* 1989;92:125–30

38. Weymuller EA Jr, Cummings CW. Cricothyroidotomy: the impact of antecedent endotracheal intubation. *Ann Otol Rhinol Laryngol* 1982;91:437–8

39. Holst M, Veress B. The healing of crico-thyroidostomy in pigs. A morphological study. *Acta Oto-Laryngol* 1989;107:300–6

40. Greisz H, Qvarnstorm O, Willien R. Elective cricothyroidotomy: a clinical and histopatho-logical study. *Crit Care Med* 1982;10:387–9

41. Sise MJ, Shackford SR, Cruickshank JC. Cricothyroidotomy for long-term tracheal access. A prospective analysis of morbidity and mortality in 76 patients. *Ann Surg* 1984;200:13–17

42. Holst M, Hertegard S, Persson A. Vocal dysfunction following cricothyroidotomy: a prospective study. *Laryngoscope* 1990;110:749–55

43. Gleeson MJ, Pearson RC, Armistead S, *et al.* Voice changes following cricothyroidotomy. *J Laryngol Otol* 1984;98:1015–19

44. Holst M, Halbig I, Persson A, *et al.* The cricothyroid muscle after cricothyroidotomy. A porcine experimental study. *Acta Oto-Laryngol* 1989;107:136–40

45. Van Hasselt EJ, Bruining HA, Hoeve LJ. Elective cricothyroidotomy. *Intensive Care Med* 1985;11:207–9

46. Cole RR, Aguilar EA 3rd. Cricothyroidotomy versus tracheotomy: an otolaryngologist's perspective. *Laryngoscope* 1988;98:131–5

47. Fisher JA. A 'last ditch' airway. *Can Anaesth Soc J* 1979;26:225–30

48. Matthews HR, Hopkinson RB. Treatment of sputum retention by minitracheotomy. *Br J Surg* 1984;71:147–50

49. Mastboom WJB, Wobbes TH, van den Dries A. Bronchial suction by minitracheotomy as an effective measure against sputum retention. *Surg Gynecol Obstet* 1991;173:187–92

50. Squires SJ, Frampton MC. The use of mini-tracheostomy and high frequency jet ventila-tion in the management of acute airway obstruction. *J Laryngol Otol* 1986;100:1199–202

51. Randell TT, Tierala EK, Lepantalo MJ, *et al.* Prophylactic minitracheostomy after thora-cotomy: a prospective, random control, clinical trial. *Eur J Surg* 1991;157:501–4

52. Clancy MJ. A study of the performance of cricothyroidotomy on cadavers using the Minitrach II. *Arch Emerg Med* 1989;6:143–5

53. Ravlo O, Bach V, Lybecker H, *et al.* A comparison between two emergency crico-thyroidotomy instruments. *Acta Anaesthesiol Scand* 1987;31:317–19

54. Au J, Walker WS, Inglis D. Percutaneous cricothyroidostomy (minitracheostomy) for bronchial toilet: results of therapeutic and prophylactic use. *Ann Thorac Surg* 1989;48:850–2

55. Buckels NJ, Khan ZH, Irwin ST, *et al.* Post-operative sputum retention treated by minitracheostomy – a ward procedure? *Br J Clin Pract* 1990;44:169–71

56. Ciaglia P, Brady C, Graniero D. Emergency percutaneous dilatational cricothyroidostomy: use of modified nasal speculum. *Am J Emerg Med* 1992;10:152–55

57. Frei FJ, Meier PY, Lang FJ, *et al.* Cricothyreotomy using the Quicktrach coniotomy instrument set. *Anasth Intensivther Notfallmed* 1990;25(Suppl 1):44–9

58. Randell T, Kalli I, Lindgren L, *et al.* Minitracheotomy: complications and follow-up with fibreoptic tracheoscopy. *Anaesthesia* 1990;45:875–9

59. Reed JP, Kemph JP, Hamelberg W, *et al.* Studies with transtracheal artificial respiration. *Anesthesiology* 1954;15:28–41

60. Bougas TP, Cook CD. Pressure–flow charac-teristics of needles suggested for transtracheal resuscitation. *N Engl J Med* 1960;262:511–13

61. Yealy DM, Plewa MC, Stewart RD. An evaluation of cannulae and oxygen sources for pediatric jet ventilation. *Am J Emerg Med* 1991;9:20–3

62. Dallen LT, Wine R, Benumof JL. Spontaneous ventilation via transtracheal large-bore intravenous catheters is possible. *Anesthesiology* 1991;75:531–3

63. Pottecher T, Bing J, Cuby C. Emergency translaryngeal ventilation with a Tuohy needle. Use in case of an inability to intubate and ventilate a curarized patient. *Ann Fr Anesth Reanim* 1984;3:54–8

64. Carden E, Becker G, Hamood H. An improved percutaneous jetting system for use during microlaryngeal operations. *Can Anaesth Soc J* 1977;24:118–25

65. Yealy DM, Stewart RD, Kaplan RM. Myths and pitfalls in emergency translaryngeal ventila-tion: correcting misimpressions. *Ann Emerg Med* 1988;17:690–2

66. Mackenzie CF, Barnas GM, Smalley J, *et al.* Low-flow endobronchial insufflation with air for 2 hours of apnea provides ventilation adequate for survival. *Anesth Analg* 1990;71:279–84

67. Frame SB, Simon JM, Kerstein MD. Percutaneous transtracheal catheter ventilation (PTCV) in complete airway obstruction – a canine model. *J Trauma* 1989;29:774–80

68. Maestracc P, Griffon H, Livrelli N. Study of pressure and EtCO$_2$ during ventilation by injection (preliminary note). *Ann Anesthesiol Fr* 1976;17:878–88

69. Slutsky AS, Watson J, Leith DE. Tracheal insufflation of O$_2$ (TRIO) at low rates sustains life for several hours. *Anesthesiology* 1985;63:278–86

70. Smith RB. Ventilation at high respiratory frequencies. High frequency positive pressure ventilation, high frequency jet ventilation and high frequency oscillation. *Anaesthesia* 1982;37:1011–18

71. Schuster DP, Karsch R, Cronin KP. Gas transport during different modes of high-frequency ventilation. *Crit Care Med* 1986;14:5–11

72. Muller WJ, Gerjarusek S, Scherer PW. Studies of wall shear and mass transfer in a large scale model of neonatal high-frequency jet ventilation. *Ann Biomed Eng* 1990;18:69–88

73. Kan AF, Gin T, Lin ES, *et al.* Factors influencing humidification in high-frequency jet ventilation. *Crit Care Med* 1990;18:537–9

74. Kovenranta H, Carlo WA, Goldthwait DA Jr. Carbon dioxide elimination during high-frequency ventilation. *J Pediatr* 1987;111:107–13

75. Jaeger MJ, Kurzweg UH, Banner MJ. Transport of gases in high-frequency ventilation. *Crit Care Med* 1984;12:708–10

76. Bourgain JL, Mortimer AJ, Sykes MK. Carbon dioxide clearance and deadspace during high frequency jet ventilation. Investigations in the dog. *Br J Anaesth* 1986;58:81–91

77. Calkins JM, Waterson CK, Quan SF, *et al.* Effect of alterations in frequency, inspiratory time, and airway pressure on gas exchange during high frequency jet ventilation in dogs with normal lungs. *Resuscitation* 1987;15:87–96

78. Sherry KM, Windsor JP, Feneck RO. Comparison of the haemodynamic effects of intermittent positive pressure ventilation with high frequency jet ventilation. Studies following valvular heart surgery. *Anaesthesia* 1987;42:1276–83

79. Fusciardi J, Rouby JJ, Benhamou D, *et al.* Hemodynamic consequences of increasing mean airway pressure during high-frequency jet ventilation. *Chest* 1984;86:30–4

80. Beamer WC, Prough DS, Royster RL, *et al.* High frequency jet ventilation produces auto-PEEP. *Crit Care Med* 1984;12:734–7

81. Otto CW, Quan SF, Conahan TJ. Hemodynamic effects of high-frequency jet ventilation. *Anesth Analg* 1983;62:298–304

82. Carlon GC, Kahn RC, Howland WS. Clinical experience with high frequency jet ventilation. *Crit Care Med* 1981;91:1–6

83. Smith RB, Babinski M, Klain M, *et al.* Percutaneous transtracheal ventilation. *J Am Coll Emerg Physicians* 1976;5:765–70

84. Jorden RC, Moore EE, Marx JA. A comparison of PTV and endotracheal ventilation in an acute trauma model. *J Trauma* 1985;25:978–83

85. Tan SS, Dhara SS, Sim CK. Removal of a laryngeal foreign body using high frequency jet ventilation. *Anaesthesia* 1991;46:741–3

86. Mackenzie CF, Barnas G, Nesbitt S. Tracheal insufflation of oxygen at low flow: capabilities and limitations. *Anesth Analg* 1990;71:684–90

87. Rone CA, Pavlin EG, Cummings CW. Studies in transtracheal ventilation catheters. *Laryngoscope* 1982;92:1259–64

88. Ward KR, Menegazzi JJ, Yealy DM, *et al.* Translaryngeal jet ventilation and end-tidal PCO$_2$ monitoring during varying degrees of upper airway obstruction. *Ann Emerg Med* 1991;20:1193–7

89. Carlon GC, Griffin J, Ray C Jr, *et al.* High frequency jet ventilation in experimental airway disruption. *Crit Care Med* 1983;11:353–5

90. Weymuller EA Jr, Pavlin EG, Paugh D. Management of difficult airway problems with percutaneous transtracheal ventilation. *Ann Otol Rhinol Laryngol* 1987;96:34–7

91. Lassa RE, Habal MB, Ross N, *et al.* Rapid access airway: surgical device and technique. *Int Surg* 1978;63:152

92. Scheinin B, Orko R, Orsback C. Ventilation through a mini-tracheostomy. An experimental study in pigs. *Ann Chir Gynaecol* 1987;76:327–9

93. Campbell CT, Harris RC, Cook MH, *et al.* A new device for emergency percutaneous transtracheal ventilation in partial and complete airway obstruction. *Ann Emerg Med* 1988;17:927–31

94. Ravussin P, Freeman P. A new transtracheal catheter for ventilation and resuscitation. *Can Anaesth Soc J* 1985;32:60–4

95. Matthews HR, Fischer BJ, Smith BE. Minitracheostomy: a new delivery system for jet ventilation. *J Thorac Cardiovasc Surg* 1986;92:673–5

96. Mammel MC, Ophoven JP, Lewallen PK, *et al.* High-frequency ventilation and tracheal injuries. *Pediatrics* 1986;77:608–13

97. Kercsmar CM, Martin RJ, Chatburn RL. Bronchoscopic findings in infants treated with high-frequency jet ventilation versus conventional ventilation. *Pediatrics* 1988;82:884–7

98. Donald PJ, Bernstein L. Subglottic hemorrhage following translaryngeal needle aspiration. Report of a case. *Arch Otolaryngol* 1975;101:395–6

99. Shuptrine JR, Auffant RA, Gal TJ. Cerebral and cardiopulmonary responses to high-frequency jet ventilation and conventional mechanical ventilation in a model of brain and lung injury. *Anesth Analg* 1984;63:1065–70

100. Wei HF, Jin SA, Bi HS. Hemodynamic effects of high frequency jet ventilation during acute hypovolemia. *J Tongji Med Univ* 1991;11:174–81

101. O'Sullivan TJ, Healy GB. Complications of Venturi jet ventilation during microlaryngeal surgery. *Arch Otolaryngol* 1985;111:127–31

102. Lindholm P, Outzen KE. Pneumothorax during jet ventilation in laryngobronchoscopy. *Ugeskrift Laeger* 1991;153:199–200

103. Kiyama S, Koyama K, Takahashi J, *et al.* Tension pneumothorax resulting in cardiac arrest during emergency intubation under transtracheal jet ventilation. *J Anesth* 1991;5:427–30

104. Bourreli B, Bigot A, Wesoluch M, *et al.* Pneumomediastinum and subcutaneous emphysema after translaryngeal jet ventilation. *Ann Fr Anesth Reanim* 1984;3:377–9

105. Egol A, Culpepper JA, Snyder JV. Barotrauma and hypotension resulting from jet ventilation in critically ill patients. *Chest* 1985;88:98–102

106. Yealy DM, Plewa MC, Reed JJ, *et al.* Manual translaryngeal jet ventilation and the risk of aspiration in a canine model. *Ann Emerg Med* 1990;19:238–41

107. O'Donnell JM, Thompson DR, Layton TR. the effect of high-frequency jet ventilation on intracranial pressure in patients with closed head injuries. *J Trauma* 1984;24:73–5

108. Marquez J, Guntupalli K, Sladen A, *et al.* Renal function and renin secretion during high frequency jet ventilation at varying levels of airway pressure. *Crit Care Med* 1983;11:930–2

109. Vesalius A. *DeHumani Corporis Fabrica Libri Septem*. Basel, 1555

110. Colles A. On stenosis of the trachea after tracheotomy for croup and diphtheria. *Ann Surg* 1886;3:499–507

111. Kato I, Uesugi K, Kikuchihara M, *et al.* Tracheostomy – the horizontal tracheal incision. *J Laryngol Otol* 1990;104:322–5

112. Price HC, Postma DS. Tracheostomy. *Ear Nose Throat J* 1983;62:447–83

113. Eliachar I, Zohar S, Golz A, *et al.* Permanent tracheostomy. *Head Neck Surg* 1984;7:99–103

114. Lulenski GC, Batsakis JG. Tracheal incision as a contributing factor to tracheal stenosis. An experimental study. *Ann Otol Rhinol Laryngol* 1975;84:781–6

115. Bercic J, Pocajt M, Drzecnik J. The influence of tracheal vascularization on the optimum location, shape and size of the tracheostomy in prolonged intubation. *Resuscitation* 1978;6:131–43

116. Fry TL, Jones RO, Fischer ND, *et al.* Comparisons of tracheostomy incisions in a pediatric model. *Ann Otol Rhinol Laryngol* 1985;94:450–3

117. Leverment JN, Milne DM. Tracheo-graft fistulae following pharyngo-laryngo-eosophagectomy. A cause and its prevention. *J Laryngol Otol* 1979;93:293–8

118. Fairshter RD, Liff MO, Wilson AF. Complications of long tracheostomy tubes. *Crit Care Med* 1976;4:271–3

119. Cane RD, Woodward C, Shapiro BA. Customizing fenestrated tracheostomy tubes: a bedside technique. *Crit Care Med* 1982;10:880–1

120. Snyder GM. Individualized placement of tracheostomy tube fenestration and *in-situ* examinations with the fiberoptic laryngoscope. *Respir Care* 1983;28:1294–8

121. Klausen NO, Lomholt N, Qvist J. Dilatation of the trachea treated with the NL-tracheostomy tube. *Crit Care Med* 1982;10:52–4

122. Dunn CR, Dunn DL, Moser KM. Determinants of tracheal injury by cuffed tracheostomy tubes. *Chest* 1974;65:128–35

123. Lomholt N, Borgeskov S, Kirkby B. A new tracheostomy tube. *Acta Anaesth Scand* 1981;25:407–11

124. Bryant LR, Trinkle JK, Dubilier L. Reappraisal of tracheal injury from cuffed tracheostomy tubes. *J Am Med Assoc* 1971;215:625–8

125. McLaughlin J, Iserson V. Emergency pediatric tracheostomy: a usable technique and model for instruction. *Ann Emerg Med* 1986;15:463–5

126. Gunawardana RH. Experience with tracheostomy in medical intensive care patients. *Postgrad Med J* 1992;68:338–41

127. Goldstein SI, Breda SD, Schneider KL. Surgical complications of bedside tracheotomy in an otolaryngology residency program. *Laryngoscope* 1987;97:1407–9

128. Hawkins ML, Burrus EP, Treat RC, *et al.* Tracheostomy in the intensive care unit: a safe alternative to the operating room. *South Med J* 1989;82:1096–8

129. Hunt JL, Purdue GF, Gunning T. Is tracheostomy warranted in the burn patient? Indications and complications. *J Burn Care Rehabil* 1986;7:492–5

130. Lesnik I, Rappaport W, Fulginiti J, *et al.* The role of early tracheostomy in blunt, multiple organ trauma. *Am Surg* 1992;58:346–9

131. Rodriguez JL, Steinberg SM, Luchetti FA, *et al.* Early tracheostomy for primary airway management in the surgical critical care setting. *Surgery* 1990;108:655–9

132. Dunham CM, LaMonica CA. Prolonged tracheal intubation in the trauma patient. *J Trauma* 1984;24:120–4

133. Desjardins R, Desjardins G, Blanc VF, *et al.* Nasotracheal intubation and tracheostomy in acute epiglottitis and laryngotracheal bronchitis. *J Otolaryngol* 1978;7:230–6

134. Lund T, Goodwin CW, McManus WF. Upper airway sequelae in burn patients requiring endotracheal intubation or tracheostomy. *Ann Surg* 1985;201:374–82

135. Rugheimer E. Long-term intubation and tracheotomy. Verhandlungen der deutschen gesellschaft fur chirurgie. *Langenbecks Arch Chir* 1990;(Suppl 2):1093–9

136. Astrachan DI, Kirchner JC, Goodwin WJ Jr. Prolonged intubation vs. tracheotomy: complications, practical and psychological considerations. *Laryngoscope* 1988;98:1165–9

137. Stock MC, Woodward GC, Shapiro BA, *et al.* Perioperative complications of elective tracheostomy in critically ill patients. *Crit Care Med* 1986;14:861–3

138. Boyd SW, Benzel EC. The role of early tracheotomy in the management of the neurosurgical patient. *Laryngoscope* 1992;102:559–62

139. Miller JD, Kapp JP. Complications of tracheostomies in neurosurgical patients. *Surg Neurol* 1984;22:186–8

140. Cooper JD, Grillo HC. The evolution of tracheal injury due to ventilatory assistance through cuffed tubes: a pathologic study. *Ann Surg* 1969;169:334–48

141. Ching NP, Ayres SM, Paegle RP, *et al.* The contribution of cuff volume and pressure in tracheostomy tube damage. *J Thorac Cardiovasc Surg* 1971;62:402–8

142. McEnirey J, Gillis J, Kilham H, *et al.* Review of intubation in severe laryngotracheo-bronchitis. *Pediatrics* 1991;87:847–53

143. Pearson FG, Goldberg M, da Silva AJ. Tracheal stenosis complicating tracheostomy with cuffed tubes. *Arch Surg* 1968;97:380–93

144. Neiderman MS, Ferranti RD, Zeigler A, *et al.* Respiratory infection complicating long-term tracheostomy. *Chest* 1984;85:39–44

145. Neiderman MS, Merrill WW, Ferranti RD, *et al.* Nutritional status and bacterial binding in the lower respiratory tract in patients with chronic tracheostomy. *Ann Intern Med* 1984;100:795–800

146. Snow N, Richardson JD, Flint LM. Management of necrotizing tracheostomy infections. *J Thorac Cardiovasc Surg* 1981;82:341–4

147. Cole AGH, Kerr JH. Paratracheal abscess after tracheostomy. *Intensive Care Med* 1983;9:345

148. Jacobs JR, Thawley SE, Abata R, *et al.* Posterior tracheal laceration: a rare complication of tracheostomy. *Laryngoscope* 1978;88:1942–6

149. Rubio PA, Sharman TL, Farrell EM. Tracheostomy tube insertion in the pretracheal fascia. *Int Surg* 1982;67(Suppl 4):418–19

150. Strauchmann U, Wagemann W. Bleeding following tracheostomy: the brachiocephalic trunk. *Entralbl Chir* 1981;106:309–16

151. Arola M, Inberg MV, Sotarauta M, *et al.* Tracheo-arterial erosion complicating tracheostomy. *Ann Chir Gynaecol* 1979;68:9–17

152. Adolfsson R, Winblad B, Ostberg Y. Survival after haemorrhage from the brachiocephalic truncus following tracheostomy. *Acta Oto-Laryngol* 1975;80:312–15

153. Moar JJ, Lello GE, Miller SD. Stomal sepsis and fatal haemorrhage following tracheostomy. *Int J Oral Maxillofac Surg* 1986;15:339–41

154. Mika H, Bumb P, Fries J. Rupture of supra-aortic neck arteries due to lesions caused by tracheal tubes. *J Laryngol Otol* 1984;98:509–17

155. Takano H, Ihara K, Sato S. Tracheo-innominate artery fistula following tracheostomy. Successful surgical management of a case. *J Cardiovasc Surg* 1989;30:860–3

156. Nunn DB, Sanchez-Salazar AA, McCullagh JM, *et al.* Trachea–innominate artery fistula following tracheostomy. Successful repair using an innominate vein graft. *Ann Thorac Surg* 1975;20:698–702

157. Wood DE, Mathisen DJ. Late complications of tracheotomy. *Clin Chest Med* 1991;12:597–609

158. Dane TEB, King EG. A prospective study of complications after tracheostomy for assisted ventilation. *Chest* 1975;67:398–404

159. Sellery GR, Worth A, Greenway RE. Late complications of prolonged tracheal intubation. *Can Anaesth Soc J* 1978;25:140–3

160. Woo P, Kelly G, Kirshner P. Airway complications in the head injured. *Laryngoscope* 1989;99:725–31

161. Hsu S, Dreisbach JN, Charlifue SW. Glottic and tracheal stenosis in spinal cord injured patients. *Paraplegia* 1987;25:136–48

162. Oeken FW. Tracheostomy – late complications and their treatment [Author's translation]. *Zentralbl Chir* 1978;103:1169–79

163. Jones JW, Reynolds M, Hewitt RL, *et al.* Tracheo-innominate artery erosion: successful surgical management of a devastating complication. *Ann Surg* 1976;184:194–204

164. Sasaki CT, Horiuchi M, Koss N. Tracheostomy – related subglottic stenosis: bacteriologic pathogenesis. *Laryngoscope* 1979;89:857–65

165. Lebowitz PW, Geller E, Andeweg SK. Endotracheal balloon cuff dilatation of

tracheostomal stenosis. *Anesthesiology* 1982; 57:323–4

166. Grillo HC, Mathisen DJ. Surgical management of tracheal strictures. *Surg Clin North Am* 1988;68:511–24

167. Rose KG. Cicatricial stenosis in the cricotracheal region. A new surgical approach. *Halls Nasen Ohrenheilkund* 1982;30:285–9

168. Anand VK, Alemar G, Warren TE. Surgical considerations in tracheal stenosis. *Laryngoscope* 1992;102:237–43

169. Golden GT, Fox JW, Edlich RF. Emergency tracheostomy. *Am J Surg* 1976;131:766

170. Ivatury R, Siegel JH, Stahl WM, *et al.* Percutaneous tracheostomy after trauma and critical illness. *J Trauma* 1992;32:133–40

171. Schachner A, Ovil Y, Sidi J, *et al.* Percutaneous tracheostomy – a new method. *Crit Care Med* 1989;17:1052–6

172. Bodenham A, Cohen A, Webster N. A clinical evaluation of the 'Rapitrach'. A bedside percutaneous tracheostomy technique. *Anaesthesia* 1992;47:332–4

173. Ciaglia P, Firsching R, Syniec C. Elective percutaneous dilatational tracheostomy. A new simple bedside procedure; preliminary report. *Chest* 1985;87:715–19

174. Leinhardt DJ, Mughal M, Bowles B, *et al.* Appraisal of percutaneous tracheostomy. *Br J Surg* 1992;79:255–8

175. Fisher EW, Howard DJ. Percutaneous tracheostomy in a head and neck unit. *J Laryngol Otol* 1992;106:625–7

176. Toye FJ, Weinstein JD. Clinical experience with percutaneous tracheostomy and cricothyroidotomy in 100 patients. *J Trauma* 1986; 26:1034–40

177. Schachner A, Ovil J, Sidi J. Rapid percutaneous tracheostomy. *Chest* 1990;98:1266–70

178. Bodenham A, Diament R, Cohen A, *et al.* Percutaneous dilational tracheostomy. A bedside procedure on the intensive care unit. *Anaesthesia* 1991;46:570–2

179. Ciaglia P, Graniero KD. Percutaneous dilatational tracheostomy. Results and long-term follow-up. *Chest* 1992;101:464–7

180. Cook PD, Callanan VI. Percutaneous dilational tracheostomy technique and experience. *Anaesth Intensive Care* 1989;17: 456–7

181. Griggs WM, Myburgh JA, Worthley LI. A prospective comparison of a percutaneous tracheostomy technique with standard surgical tracheostomy. *Intensive Care Med* 1991;17: 261–3

182. Hutchinson RC, Mitchell RD. Life-threatening complications from percutaneous dilational tracheostomy. *Crit Care Med* 1991;19:118–20

183. Bernard SA, Jones BM, Shearer WA. Percutaneous dilatational tracheostomy complicated by delayed life-threatening haemorrhage. *Aust NZ J Surg* 1992;62:152–3

184. Hazard P, Jones C, Benitone J. Comparative clinical trial of standard operative tracheostomy with percutaneous tracheostomy. *Crit Care Med* 1991;19:1018–24

185. Paul A, Marelli D, Chiu RC, *et al.* Percutaneous endoscopic tracheostomy. *Ann Thorac Surg* 1989;47:314–15

186. Marelli D, Paul A, Manolidis S. Endoscopic guided percutaneous tracheostomy: early results of a consecutive trial. *J Trauma* 1990; 30:433–5

187. Heffner JE, Miller KC, Sahn SA. Tracheostomy in the intensive care unit. *Chest* 1986;90: 269–74

188. Walls RM. Cricothyroidotomy. *Emerg Med Clin North Am* 1988;6:725–36

189. Booth RP, Brown J, Jones K. Cricothyroidotomy, a useful alternative to tracheostomy in maxillofacial surgery. *Int J Oral Maxillofac Surg* 1989;18:24–6

Index